*I would always dress and undress in the bathroom, because
I didn't want my husband to see me. That was my biggest
concern; that was my stigma. To get rid of that feeling is
terrific, because now I look at myself and I'm happy and
I don't think cancer. I look and say, "Oh, you beautiful thing."
I don't care if he sees me or not.*

*For the best testimony to breast reconstruction you should really
be talking to my husband. He says there is a big difference in
my personality from the time I had cancer to after reconstruction. Even my relationship with my husband has changed;
I enjoy sex more. He is so pleased. The kids are gone, and
I think, "Gee whiz, it's fun to run around."*

Diane, who had a mastectomy and
breast reconstruction two years
later, is one of "Eight Women
Who Tell Their Stories" in
A WOMAN'S DECISION

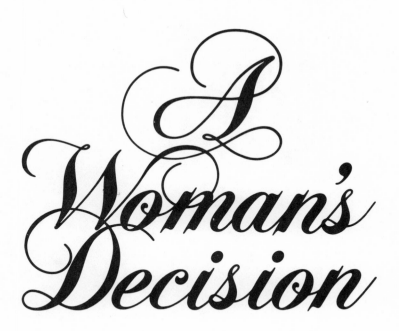

A Woman's Decision

BREAST CARE, TREATMENT, and RECONSTRUCTION

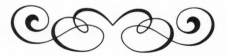

Karen Berger and John Bostwick III, M.D.

Illustrations by William Winn

BALLANTINE BOOKS • NEW YORK

Library of Congress Catalog Card Number: 85-90582

ISBN: 0-345-32485-4

This edition published by arrangement with The C.V. Mosby Company.

Manufactured in the United States of America

First Ballantine Books Edition: September 1985

10   9   8   7   6   5   4   3   2   1

CONTENTS

NOTE: THE GENDER PROBLEM

In writing this book, we were confronted with the dilemma of which gender pronouns to use to refer to the surgeons and plastic surgeons we discussed. Because all of the patients in the book are female and are referred to as she, we decided to avoid confusion and use the male pronoun for all the doctors in this book.

ACKNOWLEDGMENTS

DURING ITS DEVELOPMENT, a book progresses through many stages and numerous revisions. Though the authors may struggle in isolation committing their thoughts to paper, they need help from others to transform their rough manuscript into a published book. Assistance is required from many different sources. Our book was no exception. We were fortunate to have the advice of skilled editors, medical experts, and sensitive friends and associates. With their guidance and encouragement we worked through our problems and maintained our perspective. Therefore, we have many people to acknowledge and to thank.

The editing skills of Jeff Friedman, Carolita Deter, Sandy Gilfillan, and Fran Mues were greatly appreciated. Jeff combined his talents as writer and editor to help us focus our writing and shape and rework our manuscript. All of these talented editors read our chapters, making valuable editorial and stylistic suggestions.

A debt of special gratitude is due to Helen Crouse, who helped us to distribute 315 surveys to Reach to Recovery Volunteers in Missouri. These volunteers took time out of their lives to answer our questions because they wanted to help other women and because they had something to say. Additionally we are grateful to Ann Remington, Director of Medical Affairs, American Cancer Society, Missouri Division, who also cooperated with us in this task. Dr. Diane Fink, Vice President for Professional Education, American Cancer Society, provided another source of valuable assistance by critically reading our manuscript.

Much of the tone and focus of our book was a natural outgrowth from the emotion-packed interviews we had with the women and men who allowed us to record their feelings about and experiences with breast cancer and breast reconstruction. Particular thanks are reserved for the nine women and three men whose stories are contained within these pages. They helped us to relive their experiences with them and with our readers, and to learn from them. Even though the names and personal details of these individuals have been changed to protect their privacy, the information that remains reflects their true feelings and experiences.

Although we wrote most of this book ourselves, several chapters contain contributions from others, and we would like to acknowledge these experts here. Dr. Kenneth J. Arnold, Clinical Assistant Professor of Surgery, Washington University School of Medicine, St. Louis; Dr. John M. Bedwinek, Clinical Associate Professor of Radiation Oncology, University of Tennessee School of Medicine, Knoxville, and Director of Radiation Oncology, East Tennessee Baptist Hospital; and Dr. Gary A. Ratkin, Clinical Assistant Professor of Medicine (Hematology/Oncology), Washington University School of Medicine, St. Louis, and Chairman, Cancer Committee, Jewish Hospital of St. Louis, wrote the sections on what they do in their respective roles as general surgeon, radiotherapist, and medical oncologist, and also critically reviewed, revised, and even rewrote the information presented on these topics in Chapter 5, "Breast Cancer Facts and Treatment Options." Dr. Roger S. Foster, Jr., Director, Vermont Regional Cancer Center, and Professor of Surgery, University of Vermont School of Medicine, Burlington, carefully read and critiqued the entire manuscript and wrote the sections on clinical trials and physician-patient relations. His suggestions were enormously helpful to us. Because of contributions from these experts, our book truly provides an update on current breast cancer therapy. Other physicians provided descriptions of what they do and how they address the needs of their patients: Dr. John S. Meyer, Professor of Pathology, Washington University School of Medicine, St. Louis, and Associate Pathologist, Jewish Hospital of St. Louis; Dr. Benjamin A. Borowsky, Associate Professor of Internal Medicine, Washington University School of Medicine, St. Louis; and Dr. Jacob Klein, Assistant Professor of Clinical Obstetrics and Gynecology, Washington University School of Medicine, St. Louis. These doctors, along with Drs. Bedwinek, Ratkin, Arnold, and Foster, were enthusiastic about helping us, despite unreasonably short deadlines.

Numerous individuals have reviewed this manuscript or assisted us in gathering materials for it. Dr. Wendy Schain, National Institutes of Health, generously shared the information she had amassed, while Dr. Larry Kiel provided access to his support group for partners of women with breast cancer. Dr. Stephen Mathes, Chairman,

Department of Plastic and Reconstructive Surgery, University of Michigan Medical Center, Ann Arbor, took the time (despite a forthcoming move) to offer encouragement, review chapters, and provide suggestions. Dr. Ian Jackson, Chairman, Department of Plastic and Reconstructive Surgery, Mayo Clinic, Rochester, also critically reviewed our manuscript and contributed his comments.

This manuscript would never have been completed if it had not been for the efforts of Shirley Korn, who cared about the project and typed and retyped the manuscript because she wanted it to be right. Beth Campbell also enthusiastically participated in this effort. Their encouragement was deeply appreciated as was the cooperation and assistance of Melba Mullins, Cathy McCrary, Saundra Hayes, and Julie Baker, who effectively coordinated the Atlanta half of this endeavor.

We were fortunate to have artistic contributions from William Winn and Ann Irene Hurley, who sensitively rendered the drawings for this book. Appreciation is also due to Lester Robertson for his excellent photography.

Drs. Dean Warren, Maurice Jurkiewicz, and Waldo Powell set a standard for us; they represent the type of quality care that this book is all about. Drs. Foad Nahai, Rod Hester, Jack Coleman, and Vince Zubowicz have also been helpful through their willing efforts to assist their partner while he struggled to finish his writing. Thanks also to the plastic surgery residents at Emory.

Additional encouragement came from Drs. Eugene Courtiss, Robert Goldwyn, and Tom Rees. Dr. John H. Davis expressed his faith in this project from the first time that he learned of it. His continuing support and interest is greatly valued and appreciated.

Our friends and associates were a continual source of support, as they shared in our concerns and assisted us with our problems. Anitra Sheen and Dr. Jack Sheen not only laughed with us over our title dilemma, but Anitra provided us with napkins filled with possible choices. She and Jack were always positive and encouraging. Harriet Kopolow was the true friend that the female half of our writing team has always valued; her support was pervasive, as was Anne Hillebrandt's when she insisted on taking the manuscript home for leisurely reading. Terry Van Schaik read our book critically as both editor and friend, and her enthusiastic response was gratifying. Dr. Jessica Lewis—Jessie—was one of the reasons the book was written; it meant a great deal to know that she believed in the project and in the authors. Christine Young, despite a hectic schedule, always found time to help. She contacted potential reviewers and was a source of needed encouragement. Colleen Randall critically read the manuscript and offered suggestions. Thanks also to Marilyn Ratkin, Carol Trumbold, Pat Simons, Vicki Friedman, Jenny Mathes, and Marjorie Jackson for their friendship and assistance.

Our publishing company provided valuable support throughout this endeavor in their efforts to work with an author who was something of an anomaly, as both author and editor at the same time. Patrick Clifford, Martin Levin, Robyn Stack, Kay Kramer, Karen Edwards, and Diane Beasley gave us encouragement and assistance when we needed it most. Special thanks are reserved for Dave Danzak, who cheered us on from book conception to completion and gave us the benefit of his publishing experience.

Final appreciation belongs to our families: our spouses, Phil and Jane; our children, David and Andrew, Mary and John; and our parents, Bobbie, Paul, and Dorothy, who understood our feelings about this subject, allowed us freedom to explore them, and encouraged us in the process.

Karen Berger
John Bostwick III

A Woman's Decision

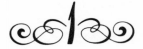

OUR PURPOSE IN WRITING

"CANCER" and "SURGERY" are words that we all have come to fear. For the woman who develops a breast malignancy, these two fears often merge when the treatment of her cancer results in the surgical removal of her breast. The idea of this operation or any operation terrifies most of us, and yet with increasing frequency, more and more women who have had mastectomies are now opting for additional, elective surgery to restore their missing breasts.

Breast reconstruction represents a major advance in the rehabilitation of women with breast cancer. Today, with the increasing emphasis on informed consent, many women stricken with this disease learn of reconstruction as an acknowledged part of their total treatment program. This was not always the case. Although techniques for rebuilding breasts have existed for many years, they were not always accepted by surgeons or known to patients. Furthermore, the results of early reconstructive efforts often did not offer sufficient aesthetic improvement to the mastectomy patient, aware of this operation, to entice her to undergo further surgery. Only recently, with the development of new procedures enabling plastic surgeons to create fuller, more lifelike breasts and to fill in major chest wall deformities, have these results improved significantly.

Despite growing acceptance of reconstruction among mastectomy patients and members of the medical community, the general public is still largely unaware of the truly remarkable physical and psychological transformation that is now possible through reconstructive breast surgery. Our book provides this knowledge in a comprehensive, but easily understandable manner. Intended primarily as a source of current and reliable information on breast reconstruction and its role in the rehabilitation of the breast cancer patient, it also focuses on a woman's options for breast care and includes routine self-inspection tips, descriptions of commonly occurring breast problems, and recent therapeutic approaches to breast cancer. Equipped with this information, women, we hope, will be able to more effectively influence their own destinies and play an active role in their own health care.

Ours is not a medical text. We are speaking as professionals, but the scope of our book extends far beyond statistical analysis or technical descriptions of tumor behavior. Rather, we incorporate the concerns of women in confronting their fears of breast malignancy and in monitoring their breasts. Our book evolved from the need for a commonsense approach to issues that women with breast problems confront in dealing with physicians and issues physicians face in treating these patients. As co-authors, we try to provide a personal, but medically accurate account.

Clearly our audience for this book is a broad one, as it should be, because breast cancer touches many people. The female half of our writing team feels that she is writing it for herself, to answer all of those questions that have always worried and haunted her. The physician half of our writing team wants to have this book to offer in answer to his patients' questions. Both of us wish to reach the one million women in the United States today who have had mastectomies and the 114,000 American women each year who develop breast cancer. We want these women to know about the option of breast reconstruction. Then women who have had mastectomies can consider this possibility, and women who develop breast cancer and choose a mastectomy (the most frequently applied therapy) can do so knowing that they can have their breasts restored. This book is also aimed at women who are disease free. If they know reconstructive breast surgery is available, they might procrastinate less in seeking medical attention for suspected breast problems. We are also writing for men, not because they will suffer from breast cancer (the incidence of breast cancer among men is 1% that of women), but because they will know, love, work with, and live among many women who have had this experience. Perhaps this knowledge will sensitize them to the psychological and physical concerns that this disease creates.

Much of the information contained within the pages of this book is drawn from 2 years of research, over 100 questionnaires, and numerous interviews with men and women. We principally surveyed women who had mastectomies for breast cancer and asked them to describe their feelings and experiences not only with this disease, but also with their subsequent therapy and rehabilitation. Of particular interest to us was information on breast reconstruction, and we posed a number of questions about this operation to determine what women knew about it and their resulting concerns and expectations for it. A sample table of contents for our book was included with the questionnaire, and we asked women to comment on the book's proposed topics and to supply us with questions that they wanted answered and issues that they wanted addressed.

In our effort to be all inclusive, our questionnaire grew lengthy, and we began to worry that no one would invest the time necessary to complete it. With the aid of Reach to Recovery and the American Cancer Society, we mailed 317 surveys to Reach to Recovery volunteers in Missouri. (These volunteers are women who have had mastectomies and, 1 year after therapy, participate in a program to bring support and information to other women in similar situations.) We received 100 responses. Moreover, the women who responded had taken a great deal of time to ponder our questions. They wrote on the backs of pages, typed extra sheets, and attached articles and reading lists that they thought would be helpful to us. As a group, they engendered important changes in the tone and direction of our book. Because of them, we have included chapters on breast self-examination, what your doctors can do for you, the man's role in the cancer experience, and selecting and communicating with your plastic surgeon.

To supplement these questionnaires, we conducted a series of taped interviews with breast reconstruction patients in different areas of the country. These women freely gave of themselves, sharing the details of their surgery, as well as their intense feelings about it. We believed that these discussions were worth preserving; consequently, Chapter 15 contains eight conversations, explaining why women seek breast reconstruction and what they can expect from it.

Although the focus of our book is not on breast disease and breast cancer, these issues are closely related to the subject of breast reconstruction. Despite the existence of numerous books and articles on the general health issues of breast disease, our survey indicates that many women remain woefully ignorant of them. Therefore, we have woven in the basic information as we go.

Still, most of our book focuses on breast reconstruction. Why do women seek breast reconstruction? Who is a candidate? What is the correct timing for this surgery? Answers to these frequently asked questions and many others are combined with the personal accounts of women who have had their breasts restored. Pain, recuperation, and expense are issues of primary concern to any woman contemplating elective surgery, and these have been dealt with in great detail. We itemize the costs, risks, and benefits and describe and illustrate the different reconstructive techniques available. We try to present all sides of this topic.

Clearly, breast reconstruction is not for every woman. Many will not wish to undergo further surgery, pain, or expense. But for those with a potential interest, we provide information to enable them to make an educated decision.

The pages that follow record the results of our efforts.

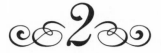

BREAST ANATOMY AND PHYSIOLOGY

HOW MUCH DO MOST WOMEN REALLY KNOW about their breasts? Most likely very little. Unless they develop breast problems, they usually are not motivated to delve beneath outward appearances to learn about the inner structure of this intimate female body part. Yet women need to be more familiar with the normal anatomy and physiology (function) of their breasts if they are going to be able to recognize the earliest and most treatable signs of breast cancer. With this knowledge, they will not be so frightened every time they notice a breast change. This chapter provides that information in a simple and straightforward manner. It offers women a baseline for evaluating their own health care requirements. Additionally, it provides assistance for women interested in performing breast self-examination, a crucial routine for proper breast surveillance.

The breast is a mound of glandular, fatty, and fibrous tissue located over the pectoralis muscles of the chest wall and attached to these muscles by fibrous strands (Cooper's ligaments). The breast itself has no muscle tissue, which is why exercises (often vigorously engaged in by teenagers intent on enlarging their breasts) will not build up the breasts. A layer of fat surrounds the breast glands and extends throughout the breast. This fatty tissue gives the breast a soft consistency and gentle, flowing contour. The actual breast is composed of fat, glands (with the capacity for milk production when stimulated by special hormones), blood vessels, milk ducts to transfer the milk from the glands to the nipples, and sensory nerves that give feeling to the breast. These nerves extend upward from the muscle layer through the breast and are highly sensitive, especially in the regions of the nipple and areola, which accounts for the sexual responsiveness of some women's breasts. Because the breast is made up of tissues with different textures, it may not have a smooth surface and often feels lumpy. This irregularity is especially notice-

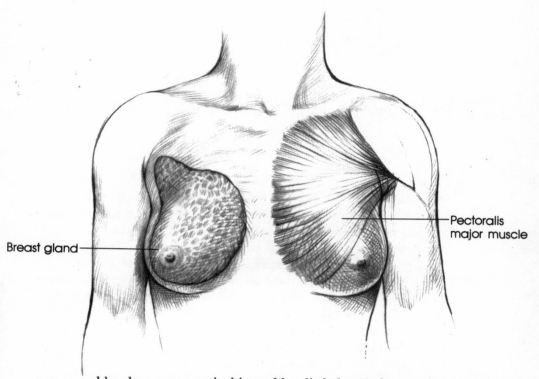

Breast gland

Pectoralis
major muscle

able when a woman is thin and has little breast fat to soften the contours; it becomes less obvious after menopause, when the cyclic changes and endocrine stimulation of the breast have ended. The breast glands drain into a collecting system of ducts at the base of the nipple. The ducts then extend through the nipple and open on its outer surface. In addition to serving as a channel for milk, the ducts are often the source of breast problems. Experts now believe that most breast cancer begins in the lining of the ducts and perhaps the milk glands. Benign fibrocystic changes also originate from these ducts.

The ducts end in the nipple, which projects from the surface of the breast, and are a conduit for the milk secreted by the glands and suckled by a baby during breast feeding. There is considerable variation in women's nipples. For some the nipple is constantly erect; in others it only becomes erect when stimulated by cold, physical contact, or sexual activity. Still other women have inverted nipples. Surrounding the nipple is a slightly raised circle of pigmented skin called the areola. The nipple and areola contain specialized muscle

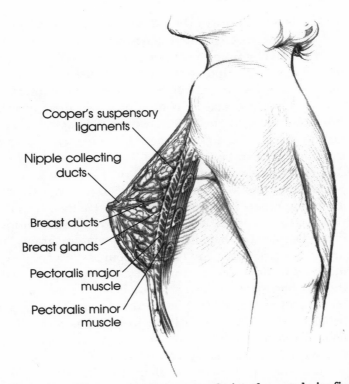

Cooper's suspensory ligaments

Nipple collecting ducts

Breast ducts

Breast glands

Pectoralis major muscle

Pectoralis minor muscle

fibers that make the nipple erect and give the areola its firm texture. The areola also contains Montgomery's glands, which may appear as small lumps on the surface of the areola. These glands lubricate the areola and are not symptoms of an abnormal condition.

Beneath the breast is a large muscle, the pectoralis major; the breast rests on this muscle, which moves the arm. Originating on the chest wall, the pectoralis major extends deep under the breast to attach on the upper arm. It also helps form the axillary fold, created where the arm and chest wall meet. The axilla (armpit) is the depression behind this fold. Removal of the pectoralis major muscle during a radical mastectomy leaves a considerable deformity: the chest has a hollowed-out appearance under the collarbone, the skin may be tight and drawn over the rib cage, and the axillary fold and axilla are missing.

A rich system of blood vessels transport and supply nutrients and hormones to the breast. Because blood flow is increased during the menstrual cycle, pregnancy, and sexual stimulation, the breasts become engorged.

Fluid leaves the breast through the venous part of the bloodstream and the lymphatic channels. The lymphatics are small vessels that carry fluid away from the breast, where it passes through a system of filters known as lymph nodes. As part of the body's immune system, the lymph nodes can enlarge in response to local infection or tumor. Trapped breast cancer cells multiplying in these lymph nodes also can cause them to swell. The two main lymph drainage areas are under the breastbone and in the axilla. Enlarged lymph nodes in the axilla usually can be felt.

In examining a woman's breasts, the physician first checks the appearance of the skin and nipple-areola for any changes, such as dimpling, nipple inversion, or crusting. He then feels the glandular tissue of the breast to detect suspicious or unusual lumps or thickenings. (Despite the beneficial value of mammograms, the physical breast examination is still the most common way of detecting breast masses.) In addition, he examines her underarm to determine if there is lymph node enlargement. When breast cancer spreads, it often can be detected first in the underarm. Thus, a patient who is being treated for breast cancer usually has some of these lymph nodes from the underarm removed and examined by a pathologist to see if the cancer has spread to them.

Each woman's breasts are shaped differently. Individual breast appearance is influenced by the volume of a woman's breast tissue and fat, her age, her heredity, the quality and elasticity of her breast skin, and the influence of breast hormones.

The breast is responsive to a complex interplay of hormones that cause the breast tissue to develop, enlarge, and produce milk. The three major hormones affecting the breast are estrogen, progesterone, and prolactin, which cause glandular tissue in both the breast and uterus to change during a woman's menstrual cycle. Because of reduced hormonal levels, the breasts are less full for 1 to 2 weeks after menstrual flow; therefore, it is easier to detect breast lumps during this time. Reduction of hormonal levels is also responsible for the breast's return to its prepregnant state after breast feeding is concluded.

Some women have a large amount of breast tissue and/or breast fat and thus have large breasts. Others have a small, but normal amount of breast tissue with little breast fat and thus have small breasts. After weight loss or pregnancy many women experience a decrease in breast size and volume. If the skin does not have sufficient elasticity, the breasts also can appear to droop or sag. The size of a woman's breasts often influences whether they will sag. The larger the breasts are, the more likely they are to succumb to the constant pressure of gravity. This sagging appearance (ptosis) often accompanies the aging process.

Few women have completely balanced breasts; one side is often larger or smaller, higher or lower or shaped differently from the other side. Breast asymmetry is normal, even though some women are not aware of it unless it is pointed out to them.

Breast shape and appearance change as a woman ages. In the young woman, the breast skin is stretched and expanded by the developing breasts. The breast in the adolescent is usually hemispherical, rounded, and equally full in all areas. As a woman gets older, the top side of the breast tissue settles to a lower position, the skin stretches, and the shape of the breast changes. After menopause, with the decrease of hormonal activity affecting and stimulating the breast, the composition of the breast changes; the amount of glandular tissue decreases and fat and ductal tissue become the predominant components of the breast. Reduction in glandular volume can result in further looseness of the breast skin.

Skin quality influences breast shape. Even though breast skin contains special elastic fibers, there is much natural and hereditary variation in the amount of elasticity and thickness of each individual's breast skin. Some women have thicker skin with considerable elasticity or stretch. They tend to have tighter and firmer breasts longer than other women who have thinner skin with less elasticity. Women with very thin skin may even develop stretch marks, or striae. These marks are actual tears of the deeper layers of the thin skin and usually indicate a lack of elasticity.

Few women realize the large area of their chest that is actually covered by breast tissue; it may extend from just below the collarbone to the level of the sixth rib and from the edge of the breastbone to the underarm area. A portion of the breast even reaches into the armpit region. The breast also has mobility on the chest wall because of loose fibrous (fascial) attachments to the underlying muscles. This breast motion is limited and the breasts are given support by special ligaments known as Cooper's ligaments. When a breast is removed, these ligaments, their fascial attachments, some lymph nodes from the armpit area, and sometimes even the underlying muscles are removed. Thus the deformity created encompasses much more than a missing breast, and for breast reconstruction to be successful, it must fill in or restore all of these areas.

BREAST SELF-EXAMINATION

BREAST SELF-EXAMINATION (BSE) can save a woman's life. Many women fear finding a breast lump and therefore avoid checking their breasts; this neglect can prove to be foolishly dangerous. It may even allow cancer to go undetected and spread outside the local breast tissue, thus lessening a woman's chances for cure and long-term survival. Periodic breast examinations are important to the early detection of breast cancer, which is the second most frequent form of cancer in women (after skin cancer). Statistics reveal that more than 90% of breast lumps are actually discovered by women themselves. If more women practiced routine BSE, the incidence of death from breast cancer might be reduced by as much as 18% because BSE-detected tumors usually are discovered when the tumor is in its earlier, more curable, stages. In addition to checking her own breasts, a woman should have her gynecologist, internist, or family physician also examine them at least once a year.

BSE is clearly an essential part of a woman's health care. It is easy to perform, does not require a special setting, and can be incorporated into any woman's normal routine. BSE helps acquaint a woman with the look and feel of her breasts and their normal cyclic changes, making it easier for her to detect breast changes early, when treatment is most likely to be effective. As a result of early detection of her breast cancer, a woman may be able to have a smaller operation.

Many women are puzzled by their breasts' natural, lumpy texture and question their ability to find a small lump within this irregular breast tissue. Initially it is difficult to differentiate between normal and abnormal breast tissue in BSE. A woman may even want to ask her doctor to help her. He can examine her breasts, tell her what he feels and why, and help her to understand what she is looking for. Eventually, with monthly inspection, she will feel more comfortable and knowledgeable about this process.

Some women have fibrocystic changes that give their breasts a lumpy texture and confound their attempts to examine themselves. These lumps frequently shrink and swell with the menstrual cycle. Women with fibrocystic disease should identify the ordinary bumpy areas of their breasts so that they can monitor cyclic changes and thus discover any new, distinct lumps.

Ideally BSE should be conducted once a month. If a woman is still menstruating, she should inspect her breasts approximately 7 to 10 days after the beginning of menstruation, when they are not swollen and tender. If she is no longer menstruating, she should still perform regular, monthly examinations; often, the first day of each month is a good, easy-to-remember time to perform this routine.

HOW TO DO BSE

BSE consists of visual and palpation (feeling) inspections.

Visual Inspection

To examine your breasts visually, stand in front of a mirror in a well-lighted room and carefully observe all sides of your breasts for anything unusual. Any differences in the size or shape of your breasts should be noted. You are looking for discharge from your nipples, sudden nipple inversion (if your nipples were previously erect), a skin rash, scaling, redness, puckering, or dimpling skin. Some women may notice that they have prominent veins in their breasts. This condition, in itself, is not cause for alarm if it is the normal state of a woman's breasts. Changes in the appearance of these veins are important. If you notice any of these variations in your breast appearance, you should immediately report them to your doctor.

To identify any changes in the shape of your breasts, observe yourself in three positions: (1) straightforward with your hands at your sides, (2) hands raised and clasped behind your head with hands pressed forward, and (3) hands pressed firmly on your hips with shoulders and elbows pulled forward. As you assume the last two positions, you should be able to feel your chest muscles tense. The outline of your breasts should have a smooth curve in all positions.

Palpation (Feeling Inspection)

The next part of the examination, feeling your breasts, can be done while you are standing or lying down. There is no need to be embar-

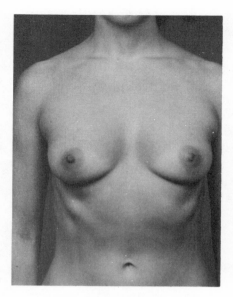

Stand straightforward with
your hands at your sides.

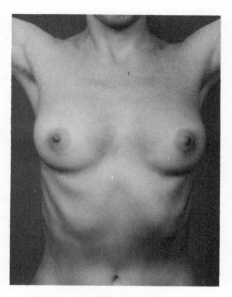

Raise your hands and clasp
them behind your head with
your hands pressed forward.

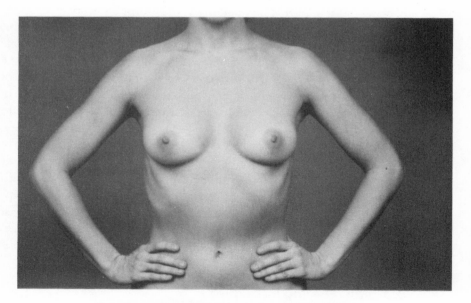

Press your hands firmly on your hips with your
shoulders and elbows pulled forward.

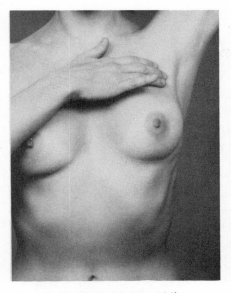

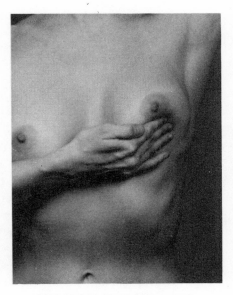

Place your fingers at the outer edge of your breast and slowly compress the breast tissue.

Move your fingers in small circles, working toward the nipple.

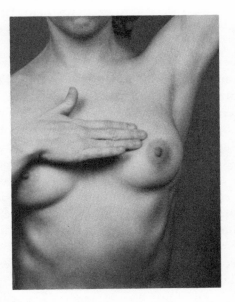

Check the entire breast and underarm, including the armpit.

rassed about feeling your breasts; this is a normal part of a woman's health care.

Many women prefer the privacy of the shower for this inspection. The soap and water make their skin feel slippery and their fingers smoothly glide over their breasts, making it easier for them to detect any textural changes underneath.

If palpation is performed while standing, begin the inspection by raising your left arm and using the flat, cushioned part of your fingers of your right hand to feel your left breast. Place your fingers at the outer edge of your breast and slowly press or compress the breast tissue gently down to the chest wall beneath. Moving your fingers in small circles around your breast, gradually work toward the nipple. Be sure to cover the entire breast and underarm, including the armpit itself. Sometimes lumps are discovered in this area. You are looking for any thickening, masses, swollen lymph nodes, or unusual lumps under the skin. They might feel like firm, distinct bumps. Repeat this examination on your right side. Women who have had a breast removed should feel their chest area, paying close attention to the scar and tissue surrounding it.

If you wish to perform the inspection while lying down, lie flat on your back with your left arm over your head and a pillow or rolled towel under your left shoulder. This position flattens your breasts and makes it easier for you to examine them. Use the same circular motion described previously and repeat the procedure on your right breast.

Remember, most women's breasts have a bumpy texture and the upper, outer portion is usually the lumpiest. The best way to discover abnormal breast lumps is to know what is normal for your breasts; then if a problem develops, you can spot it immediately. Abnormal breast lumps will vary in size, firmness, and sensitivity. They may be hard, or irregular with sharp edges. Still others appear as thickened areas with no distinct outlines. Some lumps are painful and tender. Pain is not ordinarily a sign of breast cancer, however, and may just indicate the development of a breast cyst. Sometimes, ordinary underlying anatomical structures, such as breast glands, the breastbone, or ribs, can be mistaken for lumps. Don't worry about making a mistake. Suspected lumps always should be reported to your doctor. It never hurts to be wrong, but it can definitely be damaging and even fatal to ignore a cancer.

Whether you perform BSE while standing or lying down, the important point is to make the decision to do a self-inspection each

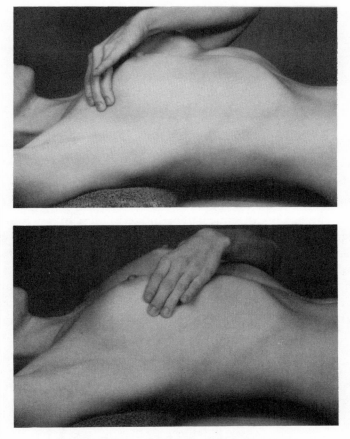

Breast self-examination while lying down.

month. Any breast changes, unusual pain or tenderness, or lumps you discover should be further investigated by your doctor. Along with your monthly BSE, you should have regular checkups by your family physician, internist, or gynecologist. A breast examination should be a routine part of this yearly office visit.

Most breast lumps are benign, but for those that are malignant, BSE and physician surveillance will ensure early detection and a significantly higher cure rate.

∝4∝

WHAT DO BREAST LUMPS MEAN?

WHEN A WOMAN DISCOVERS a breast lump, she naturally fears that she has breast cancer. Fortunately, most breast lumps are benign and are not related to breast cancer. Nevertheless, these conditions can cause a woman and her family considerable anxiety. Because of breast engorgement or inflammation, her breasts also may be painfully uncomfortable. Although many women immediately equate breast pain with cancer, most tender lumps are not malignant. Lumpy breasts, however, can be a problem and may make it difficult for a woman or her doctor to detect possible breast tumors. Awareness of commonly occurring benign breast conditions is therefore extremely valuable information for alleviating unwarranted fears and assisting a woman in early detection of a cancer if it does occur.

BENIGN BREAST CONDITIONS

Although breast cancer occurs in women of all ages, one of the important factors in predicting whether an isolated breast lump is a cancer is the person's age. Less than 3% of breast cancers occur in women under the age of 30. Most breast cancers develop after menopause. When a woman in her thirties or forties finds a lump, it is more likely to be a simple cyst filled with fluid than a cancer. Less than one third of breast cancers occur in women under the age of 50. After menopause the incidence of breast cancer rises and fewer benign breast conditions occur; thus any lump is viewed with more concern.

Fibroadenomas

When lumps are found in the breasts of teenagers and women in their twenties, they are almost always benign. The most common benign breast lump found in this age group is a firm, rounded, rub-

bery tumor known as a fibroadenoma. Fibroadenomas are not related to or precursors of breast cancer. Surgical removal is recommended for these tumors.

Fibrocystic Disease

It is normal for many women in their childbearing years to notice
that their breasts swell and become painfully tender before their
menstrual periods. Along with this swelling, the breasts often develop a lumpy texture that in some cases might become a permanent
breast characteristic. This lumpy condition is called fibrocystic disease and reflects changes within the glandular tissue and milk ducts
of the breast. Fibrocystic changes are common in women from age
20 to menopause. Because they occur during a time when a woman
has a high level of female hormones, they are believed to be related
to the response of the breast to those hormones. After menopause,
fibrocystic activity usually subsides because of a woman's reduced
hormonal level. Women taking hormones after menopause may
note a persistence of fibrocystic activity and breast fullness.

The symptoms of fibrocystic change frequently vary with a
woman's monthly cycle and are often associated with breast pain,
which may be constant or may be accentuated when her breasts are
swollen. Breast tenderness further increases a woman's anxiety that
a tumor may be present in her breast. The soreness also can prevent
a careful breast examination by the woman herself or by her physician.

Fibrocystic breasts usually feel "bumpy" with many cysts, irregu-
larities, or thickened areas; some of these lumps are indistinguish-
able from tumors. These cysts are not believed to be precancerous,
but they are noticeable breast lumps that can be confused with cancer or even obscure the diagnosis of a small cancer. Studies of large
groups of women with fibrocystic disease have demonstrated a possible link between this condition and cancer. Women with this pro-
clivity seem to be slightly more cancer susceptible.

Fibrocystic disease is usually managed without an operation. The
doctor must confirm that this is the only condition present in the
breasts. Because it is a chronic condition, it requires surveillance
over a long period by both the woman and her doctor, including
regular breast self-examination, physician follow-up and examination, mammograms (breast x-ray pictures), aspiration of cysts, and
biopsies of lumps that persist after aspiration.

In addition, some experts believe that caffeine can accentuate the
symptoms of fibrocystic disease and recommend that women with

this problem try to avoid caffeine-containing substances such as colas, coffees, teas, and chocolates. Some women notice a significant improvement after abstinence from these foods, whereas others notice no change in their breasts. Vitamin E in a daily dosage of 800 IU is believed by some to lessen the symptoms of fibrocystic disease in some women. In exceptionally severe cases, the doctor can prescribe danazol (Danocrine) to control the pain and swelling. This drug is rarely indicated, however, because it has many undesirable side effects and is extremely expensive.

Nipple Drainage

When a woman has a nipple discharge it is usually not caused by cancer. A bloody discharge, however, can indicate the presence of cancer and should never be ignored. The doctor can study a sample of the nipple discharge by spreading a thin layer of fluid on a glass slide and sending it to the pathologist for examination under the microscope.

Small, benign tumors within the nipple ducts (ductal papillomas), as well as fibrocystic changes or inflammation, can be the source of drainage. Sometimes a localized infection within a duct can cause persistent drainage. The treatment occasionally involves removal of the source of the drainage within the ductal system. The doctor also may order some hormonal studies of the blood to identify other benign causes of the nipple discharge.

DIAGNOSIS AND MANAGEMENT OF BENIGN BREAST LUMPS

Assuming that a woman finds a lump in her breast, what can she expect when she visits her doctor? The procedure varies, depending on her symptoms and her doctor's preferences. Some physicians will refer her immediately to a surgeon, whereas others might prefer to examine her first. A medical history always will be taken.

It is important to understand that referral to a general surgeon does not mean that a biopsy always will be done. Surgeons do not only cut; they are skilled in examining breast lumps, discussing and advising women about breast disease, and helping to detect and treat cancer at an early stage.

Methods for Diagnosing Breast Lumps

As a preliminary step, when a lump is first detected, the doctor or surgeon can use several noninvasive (not requiring surgery) diagnostic tools. The doctor may suggest that the woman have a mammogram (breast x-ray picture), sonogram, or thermogram. The sonogram, which uses sound waves to detect lumps, and the thermogram, which uses heat, are less specific means of detecting breast abnormalities and are thus less reliable for diagnosis. The most frequently used and reliable nonoperative diagnostic test is the mammogram. Nuclear magnetic resonance (NMR) is a new technique (not utilizing radiation) that may facilitate the diagnosis of breast cancer, thereby reducing the need for a biopsy.

Mammograms. There are two types of mammograms: conventional mammograms, which produce black and white x-ray pictures of the breast, and xeromammograms, which use a special film to produce blue and white images. Both methods are reasonably accurate in detecting breast abnormalities and provide an excellent means of finding a cancer before it can be felt and while it is still small and curable.

Unless a woman has had previous breast problems, her first mammogram should be obtained between the ages of 35 and 40 as a baseline by which to judge any future breast changes. Frequently her gynecologist or family physician will arrange for this test to help monitor her health care. After age 40, mammograms will be recommended every year or even every other year. For women considered high risk (Chapters 5 and 12) a yearly mammogram is often recommended at younger ages.

Some women fear mammograms because they worry that the radiation from the mammogram may cause the breast cancer it seeks to detect. Like any test the mammogram should be used with caution, and regular mammograms are not routinely advised for young women under the age of 35. The breasts of girls and teenagers have the highest risk of developing a radiation-induced tumor. In addition, mammograms are not as valuable in younger women because their breasts are denser, and it is more difficult to distinguish a mass or dense spot. In older women the breast tissue is less dense, and lumps are easier to identify. The radiation dosage for a mammogram is so small that the benefits of diagnosing a possible tumor far outweigh any risk of developing a breast cancer.

Breast examination and mammography are complementary diagnostic tools. Mammography alone without breast examination is inadequate; sometimes even obvious breast lumps will not show up on x-ray examination. A mammogram is a very valuable diagnostic tool, however, because it can indicate a breast abnormality at a very early stage. It cannot positively identify a mass as cancerous; this can only be done through a biopsy of the area (surgical removal of the tissue) for examination under a microscope. A biopsy is done after all appropriate diagnostic tests have been done.

When the lump in the breast feels like a cyst, it is usually drained (aspirated) with a thin needle. Occasionally, the doctor may tell the patient to return to his office after her next menstrual cycle so that he can reexamine her breast before doing needle aspiration. Tissue that shrinks and then swells again before her next cycle could be a cyst or fibroadenoma (both are benign and not related to cancer).

Needle aspiration. Needle aspiration is a method for determining if a breast mass is cystic or solid. A biopsy may be avoided if the lump disappears after the fluid has been withdrawn from the suspected cyst. Most cysts are benign; breast cancer is usually a solid tumor. The doctor may want to send the fluid for analysis to a pathologist, especially if it is blood stained. Needle aspiration is a simple and relatively painless procedure that can be done in the surgeon's office.

If the fluid is bloody or if a mass persists that cannot be aspirated, the doctor may recommend a surgical biopsy regardless of the findings on mammography. If no fluid is aspirated, the lump might be a fibroadenoma, it still might be fibrocystic disease, or it might be a cancer. Therefore, it must be investigated further to rule out the possibility of breast cancer.

In these cases, the surgeon needs to remove the lump or sample a portion of the lump to permit a specific diagnosis of the tissue by a pathologist. This sampling is called a biopsy and can be performed by needle aspiration and/or surgery.

Needle aspiration biopsy. Needle aspiration biopsy is a method of obtaining tissue by placing a needle into the tissue and removing a small sample of the breast lump for study. This method can be accurate if a good sample is obtained and the pathologist is experienced with this technique and can be certain of the diagnosis. When a benign reading is obtained, it can mean either that no abnormality is found or that the abnormal tumor was not sampled by the needle biopsy. If a suspicious lump persists after a negative needle biopsy, a surgical biopsy still may be necessary.

Surgical biopsy. A more specific and definitive procedure is known as a surgical biopsy. This method requires a small incision in the skin; the surgeon then directly identifies the lump and either removes the entire lump or a representative sample. This open biopsy is the most reliable method for obtaining a specific diagnosis of a breast lump.

When a surgical biopsy is recommended, the surgeon is concerned that the lump may be malignant. Plans must be made before the biopsy to consider the options for treatment if the lump proves cancerous. It is possible to diagnose the lump and do a mastectomy in one operation (a one-step procedure) or remove the lump and delay treatment to allow the patient time to consider her options (a two-step procedure).

If her doctor recommends a biopsy to clarify the diagnosis of her lump, a woman should ask questions about this procedure and have an explanation of it before it is performed. She should ask her doctor if he recommends a one-step or two-step procedure.

One-step procedures are requested by some women who have already decided that if they have breast cancer they prefer a mastectomy as the treatment with which they feel most comfortable. These women, having already made a decision for therapy, may select a one-step procedure to avoid the anxiety-filled interval between the diagnosis of cancer and the mastectomy to treat that disease. One-step procedures are usually done under general anesthesia. The surgeon performs the biopsy, and while the woman remains on the operating table, the tissue specimen is sent to the pathologist for a *frozen section analysis*. With this approach, the pathologist slices the tissue, quick freezes it, and stains it to permit the specific characteristics of the tissue to be identified. Through this technique the pathologist is able to make an immediate determination whether the lump is benign or malignant. This technique has the advantage of speedy diagnosis, but it is expensive and sacrifices some clarity so that occasionally the pathologist cannot make a specific diagnosis. If the report indicates that the lump is benign, the incision is closed and the woman is returned to the recovery room. If malignancy is diagnosed, the doctor will usually proceed with a mastectomy during this one-step procedure.

The two-step procedure allows a woman with breast cancer time to investigate her options and make an informed decision. She has time to obtain a second opinion and learn about the different types of therapy available for treating her cancer. In a two-step procedure, the biopsy and treatment are done at separate times. The biopsy usually can be done on an outpatient basis under local anesthesia. The pathologist then performs a "permanent section," which takes longer, but the results are easier to read than a frozen section.

With this technique, the specimen is placed in formalin (a permanent tissue preservative) and stained chemically for analysis by the pathologist. This permanent section process takes approximately 24 hours. At this time the pathologist is able to make his final report.

A woman should also ask about the length and location of the biopsy scar. Many times these scars can be short, and they can be hidden around the outer edge of the areola or placed in inconspicuous areas of the breast. Such scars often can be practically invisible once they have faded.

A woman who detects a breast lump either during self-inspection or after physician examination should constantly keep in mind the most significant fact that countless women overlook: not all lumps are cancerous. *Eighty percent of all breast lumps are benign.* She should not hesitate to have her doctor examine her and determine what needs to be done. Early detection and conclusive identification can ensure a better chance for cure if a cancer is present and can quickly alleviate a woman's needless fears if the lump is benign.

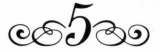

BREAST CANCER FACTS AND TREATMENT OPTIONS

BREAST CANCER TYPICALLY INVADES healthy women in their prime years. Disbelief and shock are natural responses of women faced with this shattering experience. Frequently, they are as worried about the loss of a breast as about the presence of cancer. To them "cancer" is a word, a general medical entity that strikes other people, whereas a breast is a personal and intimate body part and its loss directly threatens them in every way.

Breast cancer is the second most common cancer in American women today. Statistics from the American Cancer Society reveal that 8% of American women develop breast cancer, and it is the major cause of death from cancer for American women between the ages of 15 and 75. This year alone, over 114,000 American women will develop breast cancer. For most of these women, attempts to treat their disease and save their lives will also result in the loss of their breasts. Information about cancer, its prognosis, and the options for therapy is necessary before they can make informed and enlightened decisions about their future.

NATURAL HISTORY OF BREAST CANCER

Breast cancer most often develops in the drainage ducts of the mammary glands and is called ductal carcinoma. This is the most common type of breast cancer and occurs in 85% of the cases. In most other instances, it develops in the mammary, or milk, glands (called breast lobules) and is called lobular carcinoma. Sometimes a special type of ductal cancer, known as Paget's disease of the nipple, develops; this cancer is characterized by a rash on the nipple and an underlying small ductal cancer.

23

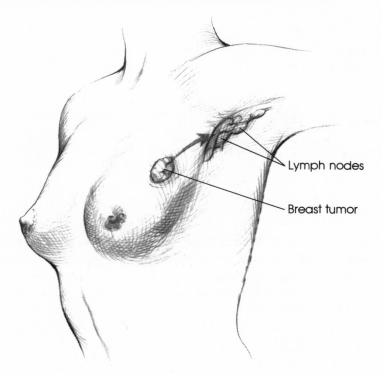

Lymph nodes

Breast tumor

Breast cancer does not appear overnight. It is not precipitated by injury or a bump to the breast. Instead, it is thought to develop as a gradual process in which certain cells lining the ducts go through a process of change from normal cells with an abnormal amount of growth (hyperplasia) to cells that are noticeably different from normal breast cells (atypical), but are not definitely cancerous. These atypical cells gradually gain the capability of growth on their own (autonomous growth), an uncontrolled growth that can extend through the cells lining the breast ducts. These cancerous cells initially grow in the breast ducts (intraductal cancer) before they spread. It is best to discover cancer when it is in an intraductal phase because it has not yet spread outside the duct lining and potentially throughout the body. When the cells of the intraductal carcinoma break through the lining outside the breast ducts, the cancer is then described as "invasive." Once the cells become invasive, they potentially can be picked up in the small lymph vessels of the breast and taken to the lymph nodes surrounding the breast, especially to those present in the armpit or beneath the breastbone. The potential also exists for invasive tumor cells to be picked up by the bloodstream and carried to other parts of the body. When tumor cells migrate to other parts of the body and continue to grow, the process is known as metastasis.

Since breast cancer develops from extremely small, microscopic cells, some experts believe that it is often present 1 to 10 years before the cancer can be felt as a mass or tumor. These tiny cancer cells have the potential to become invasive and spread to other parts of the body before the tumor can be felt, accounting for the high mortality from breast cancer and the serious nature of this disease. This invasive potential is also the reason it is so important to identify the patient at high risk and to find her breast cancer in its earliest stages, before it has a chance to spread.

RISK FACTORS

Some women are at higher risk of developing breast cancer than others. A family history, age, and previous breast cancer are three factors associated with high risk. (More information on risk factors is included in Chapter 12.)

Family history. Having first-degree relatives (mothers and sisters) who developed breast cancer increases a woman's risk by two or three times. When these relatives develop cancer in two breasts (bilateral) or they develop cancer before menopause, the risk is even greater (six to eight times or up to 50% greater).

Age. A woman's age strongly influences her risk of developing cancer. Breast cancer is unusual before age 30. The largest number of breast cancers are detected in postmenopausal women between the ages of 50 and 70 years. A third of the cases occur in patients under the age of 50 and 25% in women over 70.

Previous breast cancer. After the development of a breast cancer in one breast, the other breast is at increased risk.

BREAST CANCER STAGES

Physicians classify the spread of cancer in terms of stages. Breast cancer is graded from stage I to stage IV, and both treatment and prognosis are directly related to the stage the cancer is in when detected. Unquestionably, it is best to discover the breast cancer before stage I, in its preinvasive form, before it has spread beyond the breast ducts. Breast cancer in this preinvasive form is known as in situ cancer, and if a woman's breast tissue is removed at this stage, invasive cancer can be prevented. If no treatment is undertaken, up to 40% of these women will develop the more serious invasive cancer. Because there are various staging methods, we have not defined each of the different stages, since these definitions could prove more confusing than helpful. (See Appendix D for an example of one classification system.)

PROGNOSIS OF CANCER

The outcome, or prognosis, for a woman with breast cancer is related to the extent or spread of her disease at the time of diagnosis. Some experts believe that the size of the breast tumor affects the patient's survival. Those with small cancers, less than 1.3 cm (½ inch) in diameter, have a 20-year survival rate of 95%. Those with tumors 1.3 cm (½ inch) in diameter have an 80% survival rate, and those with 2.5 cm (1 inch) tumors have a 50% survival rate.

The lymph nodes removed during an axillary dissection provide the best prediction of the course and outcome of the tumor. The number of lymph nodes in each armpit (axillary) area varies. During an axillary dissection, usually more than half of the existing nodes are removed by the surgeon and examined by the pathologist to determine if the breast cancer has spread to this area. Patients with no involved or cancerous lymph nodes in their axilla have a 65% to 75% likelihood for survival for 10 years. If one to three nodes are found to be cancer bearing, a 40% chance exists for 10-year survival. With more than four nodes involved, less than a 20% possibility of survival is given for the next 10-year period. When any axillary nodes are involved, treatment with chemotherapy usually is recommended in an attempt to improve these chances for a more favorable outlook for the woman.

Even though these cold statistics can be quite frightening, it is important to remember that primary treatment does influence survival rates. The length and quality of life also is influenced by adjunctive treatment such as chemotherapy and radiation therapy. The use of chemotherapy for the patient with involved axillary nodes represents a significant advance in the care of cancer patients and is one method for trying to improve the prospects of those women at high risk of further spread or recurrence of their breast cancer.

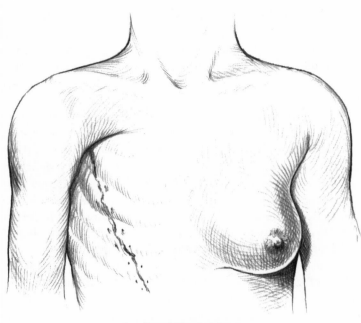

Radical Mastectomy

TREATMENT OPTIONS

PRIMARY THERAPY

Mastectomy

Today a mastectomy is the most frequently applied treatment for breast cancer. The goal of this operation is to surgically remove a woman's breast while the tumor is still in the breast area and before it has spread to other parts of her body. A mastectomy is advocated by many surgeons who believe that breast cancer is a multifocal disease in which microscopic cancers may coexist in a woman's breast with her already identified cancerous tumor. They recommend total breast removal as necessary to protect against these minute cancer cells that may remain in a woman's breast if only the invasive tumor is removed.

Several different types of surgical treatment are used for removing a woman's breast. With a radical mastectomy, the breast, underlying chest wall muscles (pectoralis major and minor muscles), and lymph glands of the armpit (axillary lymph nodes) are removed. The Halsted radical mastectomy, which was introduced 80 years ago, was the first effective operation for local control of breast cancer. Although this procedure effectively removes the breast cancer, it also leaves the woman with a large deformity. After a radical mastectomy, there is a hollowed-out area on the chest just below the collarbone, and the ribs are prominent because they are covered by a very thin layer of skin.

The mutilating aspects of the radical mastectomy and the early diagnosis of smaller breast cancers led to the development of the modified radical mastectomy. Today the modified radical mastectomy (also called total mastectomy with axillary dissection) is the method of surgical therapy chosen by most surgeons for operable breast cancer. Many surgeons believe that this operation is as effective as the radical mastectomy for controlling the breast tumor.

In this procedure the surgeon removes the breast, nipple-areola, and lymph nodes in the axilla. The lymph nodes provide further information about the spread or extent of the cancer so that the course of the tumor can be predicted. If tumor spread is evident, then appropriate adjunctive treatments such as chemotherapy, hormonal therapy, or radiation therapy can be chosen. The largest chest wall muscle, the pectoralis major, remains intact. This muscle is located in the front of the chest and helps to support the breasts; preservation of this muscle greatly reduces the deformity resulting from this mastectomy.

After a modified radical mastectomy, the chest wall will not have a hollowed-out appearance, and the ribs will still be covered by muscle and therefore will not seem overly prominent. The loss of the breast and nipple will result in a flatness to the chest. A scar will extend horizontally or diagonally across the chest. In addition, the area of the mastectomy is usually numb because the nerves that supply sensation to the chest and breast were threaded through the breast tissue which is now gone. The inside of the upper arm is also numb because the nerve to this area goes through the axillary region and is removed with the axillary dissection. After the mastectomy the armpit is usually deeper, and many women notice less perspiration on that side than on the other normal side. Because the operation extends beneath the upper arm into the axilla, the woman may experience temporary pain after the operation when she moves her arm. The general surgeon usually will recommend postoperative exercises to ensure the return of full use and function of the arm.

Today many surgeons who recommend a mastectomy for women with breast cancer also inform them of the option of breast recon-

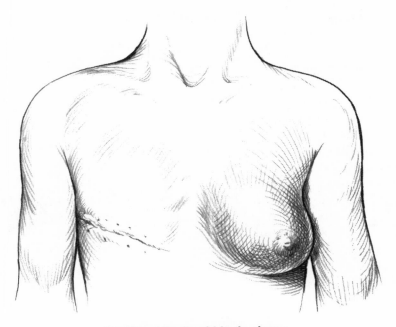

Modified Radical Mastectomy

struction to rebuild their breasts and fill in the defects left from their cancer surgery. Current reconstructive techniques allow plastic surgeons to reconstruct the deformities remaining after radical and modified radical mastectomies.

Increasingly general surgeons are cooperating with plastic surgeons to perform immediate breast reconstructions for their patients. With this procedure, women have their mastectomies and their breasts rebuilt during one operation. This approach requires teamwork between the general surgeon and the plastic surgeon. It is a viable alternative for some women because it combines the most proven and accepted treatment for their breast cancer with the immediate restoration of their breasts.

Breast Conserving Surgery and Irradiation
JOHN BEDWINEK, M.D.

An alternative to mastectomy that is used with increasing frequency is a procedure called "breast conserving surgery and irradiation." With this approach, the surgeon removes only the tumor itself or the tumor plus a margin of surrounding normal breast tissue. If only the tumor is removed, it is called a lumpectomy or tumorec-

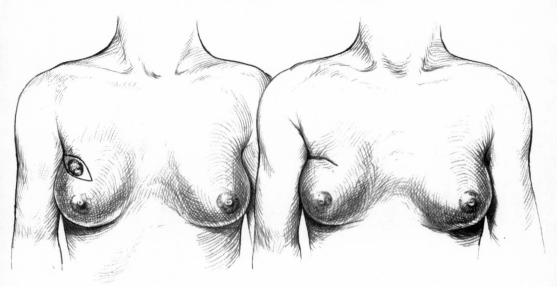

Lumpectomy

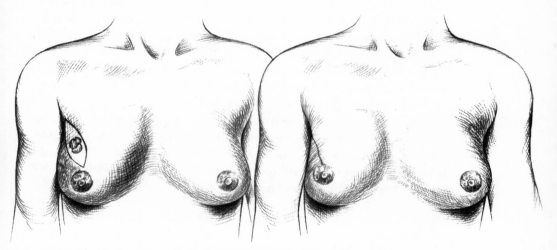

Quadrantectomy

tomy; the terms used for the removal of the tumor plus surrounding breast tissue are partial mastectomy, segmental mastectomy, or quadrantectomy. The aesthetic result with a lumpectomy is sometimes better than that achieved with a partial mastectomy, which removes a larger amount of breast tissue.

In addition to the lumpectomy or partial mastectomy, an axillary node dissection (removal of the lymph nodes under the arm) is also required. The breast is then treated with irradiation (usually about 5000 rads). After certain types of local surgery the patient may also require a boost of radiation to the site of tumor removal. This boost will either be administered with electron beams of appropriate energy externally applied at 1000 to 1500 rads or with hollow needles containing implants of radioactive material, internally placed in the breast and supplying a boost of 1500 to 2500 rads. It is important to remember that this alternative to mastectomy does not, as the title of this section implies, involve irradiation *instead* of surgery, rather it is an integration of both surgery *and* irradiation. The term primary irradiation, which this procedure is frequently called, is really a misnomer. A much more appropriate name is breast conserving surgery and irradiation, and this is the term that will be used throughout this section.

The irradiation associated with breast conserving surgery takes approximately 5 to 6 weeks to complete (one treatment each day, 5 days each week). The boost takes 1 to 6 days. It does not cause hair loss, nausea, or significant loss of energy; it will, however, cause a temporary reddening of the breast skin, similar to a mild sunburn. This reddening of the skin usually occurs 3 to 4 weeks after the beginning of the irradiation and completely disappears within 2 to 3 weeks after completion of therapy. The irradiated breast ultimately can appear and feel quite normal, provided that the irradiation is properly applied and the breast is not excessively large.

Most of the recent reports of breast conserving surgery and irradiation (particularly those involving patients who have been observed for a minimum of 10 years after such treatment) suggest that, for early breast cancer (stages I and II), this procedure is as effective as a mastectomy. Despite these reports, there is still controversy among physicians in this country regarding the equivalence of these two procedures. The patient seeking information about breast conserving surgery and irradiation will get a different opinion, depending on which physician she talks to. Many surgeons in the United States still believe that this breast saving procedure has not yet been satisfactorily proven as effective as a mastectomy. Those surgeons and radiation oncologists who do regard breast conserving surgery and irradiation as an acceptable alternative to a mastectomy regard it as appropriate only for a select group of patients. Therefore, not all women are candidates for this approach, and a woman's suitability must be determined by both the surgeon and radiation oncologist rather than by only one or the other. The following are the factors to consider in making this decision:

1. *Tumor size*. The smaller the size of the tumor, the less chance there is of a local recurrence (regrowth of tumor within the breast) after breast conserving surgery and irradiation. Most radiation oncologists do not advise this approach unless the tumor is 3 cm (1.25 inches) or smaller.

2. *Breast size*. If the breast is very small, complete removal of the tumor may leave a significant surgical defect that will mar the aesthetic result. A woman with very small breasts probably would be better off, from an aesthetic standpoint, to have a mastectomy and subsequent reconstruction rather than breast conserving surgery and irradiation. The opposite extreme, a very large breast, is also a factor in the cosmetic outcome. A very large, pendulous, and fatty breast tends to shrink after 5000 rads of irradiation; whereas a moderate-sized breast usually does not. Since a certain amount of breast shrinkage (and hence some asymmetry between the treated and the untreated breast) may still be more acceptable to a woman than having no breast at all, women with large, pendulous breasts can be considered as candidates for breast conserving surgery and irradiation. Occasionally, a woman will have breasts that are so huge that the irradiation can be technically very difficult or even impossible. Obviously such a woman should be treated with a mastectomy.

3. *The mammogram*. All women should have mammograms to ensure that there are no tiny, undetected cancers within the breast in addition to the main tumor itself. If there is a suspicion of a second undetected cancer within the breast, the woman definitely should be treated by a mastectomy.

4. *Patient attitude*. The woman must have a very strong desire to preserve both of her own natural breasts. Some women may seek breast conserving surgery and irradiation because they think this approach will eliminate the need for major surgery. This is not the case, since the tumor excision and axillary node

dissection involved in this approach constitute major surgery and will entail a recuperative period that is just about as long as that encountered with a mastectomy. The appropriate motivation for breast conserving surgery and irradiation should be a very strong abhorrence of breast loss, *not* the fear of major surgery.

5. *Physician expertise.* Whether breast conserving surgery and irradiation is a viable option should depend on the availability of a surgeon and radiation oncologist who are experienced in performing this procedure. Both the surgical and radiotherapeutic aspects of breast conserving surgery and irradiation require expertise; serious mistakes can be made if the surgeon and radiation oncologist do not know how to avoid some of the potential pitfalls. A woman may be better off to have a mastectomy than to have breast conserving surgery and irradiation by a surgeon and radiation oncologist who have only limited experience in this procedure.

A WOMAN'S OPTIONS

Today women with breast cancer have a number of options to choose from for primary treatment of their disease. Mastectomies followed by breast reconstruction and breast conserving surgery with irradiation are both positive therapeutic responses to women's expectations or requests for cancer treatment without permanent breast loss.

ADJUVANT THERAPY
Adjuvant Irradiation
JOHN BEDWINEK, M.D.

In the past, women who had mastectomies and were found to have positive axillary lymph nodes were given irradiation after surgery. The irradiation was directed to the chest wall and to the lymph nodes above the collarbone and beneath the breastbone. It was thought that this postoperative irradiation would improve survival by killing any cancer cells not removed by the mastectomy. The irradiation does, indeed, drastically reduce the likelihood of a local recurrence; that is, the reappearance of cancer on the chest wall or in the nearby lymph nodes. This prevention of a local recurrence does not seem to improve the chances of cure, however, since most patients who have a local recurrence of cancer after a mastectomy also will develop distant metastases that the irradiation does *not* prevent. Many studies have been conducted to test whether postoperative radiation will improve survival, and none of them have conclusively proven that it will.

Since today we no longer believe that combining irradiation with a mastectomy will improve the chances of cure, it is given only to those women whose chance of a local recurrence is high. These women have very large breast tumors (5 cm; 2 inches or more), enlarged lymph nodes under the arm, or tumors that have invaded into the skin of the breast or into the pectoralis muscle underlying the breast. For these patients, keeping the risk of local recurrence minimal by adding irradiation is of definite benefit because a local recurrence is difficult to treat successfully and can cause unpleasant symptoms such as pain or bleeding. Fortunately, the majority of patients who have a mastectomy today do not have a high risk of local recurrence, and postoperative irradiation is not usually needed.

Adjuvant Chemotherapy
GARY A. RATKIN, M.D.

Chemotherapy, or the use of drugs that can kill cancer cells allowing the normal tissues to heal and recover normal functions, has been a major advance in cancer management. This is the newest form of treatment available for breast cancer. Adjuvant chemotherapy involves the use of drugs that attempt to destroy breast cancer cells when they are present in a microscopic form outside of the breast. When a patient is at high risk of distant spread of the cancer, because the axillary lymph nodes are involved, adjuvant chemotherapy is now advised as a preventive measure. This therapy is used in conjunction with a mastectomy or with breast conserving surgery and irradiation.

Most chemotherapy is administered intravenously. Few agents are available in pill form. Based on the use of chemotherapy to control advanced cases of breast cancer ("palliative" chemotherapy), the oncologist now uses combinations of effective drugs for many women to attempt to lower the risk of recurrence. These drugs usually are administered in brief courses given every 3 or 4 weeks. Some of the most frequently used medications include melphalan (Alkeran), methotrexate, 5-fluorouracil, cyclophosphamide, vincristine, and prednisone. Today, three or more of these medications may be used in combination.

Although they are used to try to improve a woman's prognosis, these chemotherapy drugs can cause temporary side effects, including nausea, vomiting, hair loss, low blood cell counts, low platelet counts, interruption of the menstrual cycle, and fatigue. Fortunately, much has been learned about the ways of reducing or preventing some of these side effects. For instance, nausea is treatable and often totally preventable. Even hair loss, which is a widely publicized side effect of chemotherapy, does not happen with every drug and can be avoided in up to 50% of patients who receive a drug such as doxorubicin (Adriamycin) (known to cause hair loss in most patients) by the use of a scalp-cooling device.

An important type of chemotherapy toxicity is the lowering of white, red, or platelet blood counts that may occur 1 to 3 weeks after most programs. This side effect of chemotherapy is usually short lived and is not serious unless the patient develops an infection because of the lowered resistance resulting from a low white blood count. Similarly, bleeding is an unusual complication of chemotherapy caused by a low platelet count. For this reason blood counts are carefully monitored before and frequently between courses of chemotherapy.

Other side effects such as mouth sores, diarrhea, fatigue, and bladder irritation are related to specific drugs that may be administered. These side effects often can be prevented, and patients are informed of the potential complications and the means to avoid these problems.

Encouraging results are now being reported for preventive chemotherapy programs that are given for 6 to 12 months after cancer diagnosis and treatment. These results demonstrate that some women with axillary node involvement who receive chemotherapy live longer than those who did not receive chemotherapy.

If Breast Cancer Spreads . . .
GARY A. RATKIN, M.D.

If the primary and adjunctive therapies are not totally effective in eradicating all disease, the cancer may return at some future date. Patients with breast cancer are followed up carefully by their physicians to maintain vigilance for potential recurrence. Although the chance of cure is not always possible once a recurrence is found, the patient may have many years of functional, good-quality life with treatment. Breast cancer, unlike many other forms of metastatic cancer, can be well controlled for long periods of time with the use of medications or surgical techniques. Recently, much progress has been made in the treatment of such widespread breast cancer.

Hormonal Therapy
GARY A. RATKIN, M.D.

By altering the patient's hormonal balance, the physician can some-times effectively treat her breast cancer when it has relapsed or spread. Today, female hormone receptors (estrogen and proges-terone) can be detected and measured in most breast tumors; their presence indicates whether the tumor is likely to be responsive to hormonal treatment, which attempts to manipulate the stimulating effect of estrogen and progesterone on tumor growth. The presence of hormone receptors also predicts a better prognosis for the patient. If the cancer returns or spreads outside of the breast, the hormone receptor test predicts which patients will respond to this therapy.

By properly applying hormonal therapy to women who have hor-mone receptors, the chance of a response to hormonal therapy for the patient with advanced breast cancer is greater than 50%. These hormonal responses may last for a year or longer. Women who re-spond to one form of hormonal manipulation have a good chance of subsequent responses. Negative hormone receptors on the initial test of a breast specimen or a later biopsy predict a less than 10% chance of response to hormonal types of treatment.

Hormonal therapy can take several forms. A woman who is still having menstrual periods might benefit from an oophorectomy, an operation to remove her ovaries, the primary source of estrogen in her body. Some women have profited from the eventual removal of the adrenal glands or pituitary gland to further prolong a hormonal response.

More commonly today, medical forms of hormonal therapy are used rather than surgical removal of a hormone-producing gland. An antiestrogen, tamoxifen (Nolvadex), can be effective in selected patients in both the premenopausal and postmenopausal groups of women. Generally, this drug has only a few side effects that resemble menopausal symptoms; however, some patients will have lowered white blood and platelet counts.

Estrogen in medication form is used in women after menopause. Such conjugated estrogen preparations as Premarin or diethylstil-bestrol in relatively high therapeutic doses can be as effective as tamoxifen but can produce more frequent side effects such as nausea, swollen ankles, or engorgement of the breast. Another "female" hormone that can be effective in widespread breast cancer is the use of a large dose of progestational hormone such as megestrol acetate (Megace) or medroxyprogesterone (Provera). Side effects for progestational hormones are an increase in appetite and weight. A male hormone preparation known as an androgen, used in the past, has been largely abandoned because it causes fluid retention and has masculinizing effects (facial and body hair, deepening voice). More recently a new drug known as aminoglutethimide (Cytadren) has been introduced; this drug is effective as a form of hormone suppression. The use of aminoglutethimide allows the physician to temporarily block adrenal gland function and thus accomplish the same effect as was achieved previously with surgical removal of the adrenal glands. This agent does have the risk of inducing a severe skin rash, initial drowsiness, chemical imbalance due to the lack of adrenal hormones, and nausea in the patient.

CHEMOTHERAPY FOR WIDESPREAD DISEASE
GARY A. RATKIN, M.D.

Today, chemotherapy can be effectively applied in the woman whose breast cancer has recurred locally, metastasized, or spread widely throughout her body, involving other organs such as the lungs, liver, or bone marrow. In general these women are believed to have a very low chance of response to hormonal therapy or are so ill that hormonal therapy will not be sufficiently rapid or potent to deal with their illness. As discussed earlier in this chapter, these drugs are frequently given in combination to produce the best chance for response in the patient.

CLINICAL TRIALS: THEIR ROLE IN ASSESSING BREAST CANCER TREATMENT OPTIONS
ROGER S. FOSTER, JR., M.D.

In the past, and sometimes even now, new treatments for breast cancer are introduced without first receiving the scientific scrutiny necessary to establish their value. Before these treatments are accepted by the medical community for use with patients, they need to be compared to alternative treatments in carefully conducted scientific studies.

The randomized clinical trial represents an excellent method for comparing and assessing different treatment approaches to breast cancer management. In these clinical trials, groups of doctors and their women patients agree to participate in studies in which the cancer treatment alternatives that these patients will ultimately receive are decided by randomization. Randomization means that neither the patient nor her doctor chooses between the alternative treatments; instead the treatments are chosen arbitrarily, or totally by chance, to avoid any bias creeping into the study. Randomized studies are particularly important when the differences between treatments being compared are likely to be either small or nonexistent.

These clinical trials now involve thousands of women whose medical data have been carefully collected to answer a variety of scientific questions about breast cancer. Out of these trials has come an understanding that breast cancer is not one disease but many different diseases, or perhaps a disease with many variations. Increasingly, appropriate treatment requires understanding these many variations of breast cancer.

Primary Treatment: Partial versus Total Mastectomy

The treatment of breast cancer by less than complete mastectomy is currently being studied in randomized clinical trials. Two important trials recently completed in this area contribute significantly to resolving questions that were unsatisfactorily answered previously. More time will be necessary for answers on long-term outcome, but it appears that when carefully selected patients are treated by experienced surgeons and radiotherapists with breast conserving operations, their survival at 5 years is comparable to the 5-year survival for women treated with operations that remove the entire breast. Some partial mastectomy patients do, however, have further occurrence of cancer in the remaining portion of their breast and require a total mastectomy at a later time. As further data develop from these studies, women and their physicians will have additional scientific information on which to base a decision regarding the alternatives of total mastectomy followed by reconstruction versus breast conserving surgery.

Adjuvant Treatment

Alternative adjuvant management approaches for breast cancer have also been the subject of investigation. For many years, irradiation treatment was given after radical or modified radical mastectomy in the hope of improving the cure rate. Now, scientifically valid studies on irradiation treatment have been conducted and demonstrate that the addition of irradiation only decreases recurrence in the treated area and has no benefit on survival. We have learned that irradiation treatment is best reserved for those mastectomy patients in whom cancer recurs.

Other randomized clinical trials have investigated the question of alternative treatments for the axillary lymph nodes. These studies have shown that the axillary nodes can be treated by either surgery or irradiation with similar results. If the axillary nodes are not enlarged, they may even be simply watched and treated only if they enlarge. These studies, which were conducted more than 10 years ago, proved that treating the axillary lymph nodes does not harm any immune response the patient may be having to her cancer. Today, for most patients diagnosed with breast cancer, the axillary lymph nodes are routinely removed because up to 4 out of 10 patients will have microscopic spread of cancer into the lymph nodes, and that information is important in making decisions on additional treatments such as chemotherapy or hormonal therapy.

Randomized clinical trials have been important in studying the effectiveness of combining systemic treatments (those affecting the entire body) with local and regional treatments of irradiation and surgery. Over the past 10 years these randomized trials have been conducted to assess the effectiveness of systemic treatment with chemotherapy and/or hormonal therapy. The studies have clearly shown that, by using these adjuvant treatments, it is possible to decrease the recurrence rates and improve survival for some types of breast cancer.

Most breast cancer clinical trials require cooperation from physicians in many different medical centers. Numerous experts contribute to the design of each trial, thus providing "multiple second opinions." The National Cancer Institute reviews each trial design and commonly covers the expenses incurred in collecting the scientific data. In addition, each participating medical center has its own human investigation review committee that must approve the trial before it can begin at a medical center.

By participating in clinical trials, physicians are able to keep current with the most recent developments in cancer treatments, and patients can expect to receive either the best recognized treatment or a new treatment that a consensus of experts believes may represent an advance. In addition, information gained from the treatment will influence the future care of others.

CLOSING THOUGHTS

The feelings of attachment a woman has about her breasts are profound and should not be overlooked by the physician treating her.

These feelings will influence a woman's decision to seek help initially and eventually will help determine the type of therapy that she selects. Once the surprise of being stricken by a dreaded disease has passed, a woman desires and deserves honest information about her disease, her prognosis, and her options for treatment. In addition, she wants a physician who is sensitive to her psychological and aesthetic concerns. The physician who treats a woman afflicted with breast cancer must consider the relationship of therapy to ultimate survival, rehabilitation, and enhanced quality of life. To consider only management of her cancer is no longer sufficient.

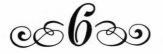

WHAT YOUR DOCTORS CAN DO FOR YOU

TODAY WE LIVE in an age of specialization. Nowhere is this phenomenon more obvious than in the field of medicine, where a single individual is no longer capable of being current with all there is to know. Thus, when a woman has a breast problem, she may consult with several experts before she can decide on the appropriate course of action. Most likely she will begin by visiting with her primary care doctor, who is familiar with her medical history and whom she has grown to trust for advice about her health care. This doctor may be her gynecologist, family practitioner or internist, and he is the person she will see for a diagnosis of her problem and treatment advice. This doctor also will refer her to other specialists if he feels that they can contribute to the diagnosis or treatment of her suspected problem. When her doctor sends her to another specialist, he is not losing interest in her case, rather he is playing an important coordinating role by using his knowledge and taking advantage of recent developments in medicine to help her get the best care possible.

A woman's needs, of course, will vary with her individual situation. Sometimes her breast problem will be diagnosed as a fibrocystic change by her primary care physician, and he will monitor her health with regular checkups and mammograms. If he finds a lump, or another problem warrants further investigation, she may be referred to a general surgeon for further examination.

If a biopsy is indicated, the story becomes even more complicated because a pathologist now becomes involved in the woman's health care. He analyzes the biopsy specimen and reports whether a cancer has been found, what kind it is, and whether it has spread to her lymph nodes. Even though the pathologist has no direct contact with the woman breast cancer victim, or even with the woman whose

41

biopsied lump proves benign, his report has a great influence on what happens to each of these women in the future. If the pathologist's report indicates cancer, then the general surgeon provides the woman with an explanation of her problem and some understanding of her treatment options. (See Chapter 5.) These options may include a mastectomy, with the possibility for breast reconstruction, or breast conserving surgery and irradiation. If cancer has spread to her lymph nodes, adjunctive therapy also may be required, and she may learn of chemotherapy, radiation therapy, and hormonal therapy. Depending on her individual situation and the therapy she ultimately selects, she may interact with a number of specialists associated with the breast management team; these experts would include the radiation oncologist (radiotherapist), medical oncologist (chemotherapist), general surgeon, and plastic surgeon.

The thought of facing more than one doctor is often a frightening one. We don't adequately understand what each of these specialists does, and it seems like an impersonal and expensive approach to health care. Furthermore, we don't always know what questions to ask these doctors or even how they can really help us. To clear up some of the confusion and impersonality surrounding these medical specialists, we have asked experts whom we know and respect in each of the previously mentioned fields to write descriptions of what they do and how they can help you. The descriptions are organized according to the role these physicians play in a woman's health care and the stage at which she might consult with each expert. Therefore, the gynecologist and internist are included under a heading entitled Primary Care: Diagnosis, Management, and Referral, and the general surgeon, pathologist, radiation oncologist, medical oncologist, and plastic surgeon are listed under The Breast Management Team: Diagnosis, Treatment, and Rehabilitation.

The nurse's role is not discussed separately in this chapter. When a woman has a breast problem, she is usually referred directly to a physician. The nurse, however, is active in all phases of the woman's breast care and plays a valuable part in patient education, therapy, and rehabilitation.

All of the specialists listed are board-certified members of their specialties. We feel that it is important for a woman to choose a physician who has met this standard. All physicians can practice medicine after medical school or residency, but having board certification indicates that after training and an initial period of practice, they have passed an examination which tests their competence and shows that they meet the criteria for practice in the specialty.

PRIMARY CARE: DIAGNOSIS, MANAGEMENT, AND REFERRAL

A yearly visit to the obstetrician-gynecologist or internist is routine for many women. If they develop a breast problem, they look to one of these doctors for advice and help.

The Obstetrician-Gynecologist's Role in a Woman's Breast Care
JACOB KLEIN, M.D.

Specializing in the care of women and their reproductive organs, the obstetrician-gynecologist is in reality the primary care physician for most women and frequently is the only doctor that they see on a regular, ongoing basis. During a woman's annual or semi-annual visits to her gynecologist, he performs physical examinations that include a breast examination, pelvic examination, and Pap smear, which is a screening test for cervical cancer.

In the absence of breast disease, the gynecologist is usually the physician who orders breast screening tests. It is his responsibility to be knowledgeable about the types of tests available, their advantages and disadvantages, and the frequency with which these examinations should be given. The newest developments in the area of breast screening must be part of every gynecologist's fund of knowledge.

The gynecologist is frequently the person most responsible for educating his patients about their bodies. This education includes information about the normal structure and function of their reproductive organs and what happens when these organs malfunction. In addition, it is the role of the gynecologist to stress the value of regular gynecological examinations and the importance of breast self-examination for early detection of breast cancer.

It is vital for the gynecologist to educate patients about the need for regular, monthly breast self-examination, as well as the best timing for these inspections. Because a woman's hormonal cycle has a profound influence on her breast tissue, she needs to understand these cyclic changes in order to know when to examine her breasts. Women have numerous reasons for not performing this test, including fear of discovering a mass, ignorance of inspection techniques or the importance of early diagnosis, and lack of awareness of the prevalence of breast cancer. The gynecologist needs to be sensitive to a woman's concerns and aware of her reasons for procrastinating about performing this health routine. With these reasons in mind, he should take responsibility for actually teaching his patients the appropriate techniques for breast self-inspection, and then he should monitor a woman's performance to make sure that her inspections are adequate and to help her gain confidence in her ability to successfully practice self-examination. He also can assure her that she will gain proficiency with this inspection if she makes it a monthly routine.

When a woman discovers a questionable breast mass, the gynecologist is usually the first physician she contacts. The relationship that exists between a woman and her gynecologist is a unique and particularly trusting one. It allows the physician to deal with the physical and psychological aspects of a woman's breast disease. Therefore, a gynecologist must sensitively respond to the patient's breast problem, from a total perspective, realizing that the discovery of a breast mass provokes unparalleled fear and anxiety in most women. The stress caused by the discovery of a breast lump must be dealt with, as well as the treatment for the actual breast problem.

The process leading to definitive treatment of a suspected breast problem is initiated by the gynecologist with a routine breast examination. His findings will either reassure him that a disease state does not exist or cause him to further evaluate the breast mass. The gynecologist will direct this evaluation by arranging for breast cyst aspiration, mammograms, or referral to a surgeon who is familiar with and sensitive to the issues involved with treating breast diseases. The patient will rely on her gynecologist for direction in her health care and will expect him to provide her with an explanation of the course of events that will probably follow.

Once evaluation of her breast problem is complete and definitive treatment planned, a woman will frequently need to be reassured by her gynecologist that the other specialist's approach is medically sound. At this time, the gynecologist plays an important role as a reliable source of information. He will continue the relationship with the patient concomitant with the care being provided to her by the surgeon, oncologist, radiotherapist, or plastic surgeon.

Prevention of breast disease and treatment of pathological breast conditions when they do occur are an integral part of routine gynecological care and should be expected and demanded by every patient.

The Internist's Role in a Woman's Breast Care
BENJAMIN A. BOROWSKY, M.D.

In current medical practice, the internist is the specialist responsible for the comprehensive medical care of his patients and the monitoring of their ongoing health care needs. His involvement in the treatment of a woman with a breast problem or breast cancer is continuous, beginning before the disease is detected and continuing after treatment is complete.

As part of health maintenance counseling, the internist will advise women on the need for self-examination and physician examination, appropriate use of mammograms, and effects of various drugs and hormones on her breasts. As more data become available on the influence of diet and environment on the incidence of breast cancer, he will discuss this information with her as well. In short, the internist's first duty is to educate the patient about practices that will prevent cancer when possible and lead to prompt detection when it does occur.

Once a breast mass has been discovered, the internist's first effort is to confirm its presence by examination. He must then choose from several options. If he feels certain that there is no indication of malignancy, he may decide not to proceed further. Repeat examination at a more suitable time in the menstrual cycle may be needed. In some cases, the use of mammography is helpful. If he is uncertain about diagnosis, he may wish to refer the patient to a surgeon for another opinion or for a biopsy and/or definitive surgery.

In selecting a general surgeon for patient referral, the internist is guided by more than the surgeon's technical knowledge and skills. He must also consider how the individual woman will relate to a particular surgeon. Each person differs in the extent she desires to be informed about the many surgical options now available. Some women (and their families) wish to play an active role in planning treatment, whereas others prefer not to have to make a choice. It is important for the internist, who usually knows the patient best, to consider her preferences in recommending a surgeon for her. It is also his responsibility to advise the surgeon as to the woman's feelings. The surgeon usually will be the source of technical information regarding the woman's surgical options, but the internist can help her and her family understand these options and can offer his advice when a choice of treatment is available.

During and immediately after surgery, the internist manages any other coexisting conditions a patient may have. He also will participate in decisions regarding postoperative x-ray treatment or chemotherapy.

After the initial therapy is complete, follow-up is a coordinated effort between the surgeon, internist, and oncologist and/or radiotherapist, when the latter are needed. It is usually the internist who carries out long-term follow-up and performs appropriate examinations to screen for signs of recurrent cancer. He also tailors his management of subsequent complaints to consider the effect treatment may have on the woman's breast cancer.

The internist functions initially in the areas of prevention and detection. After cancer has been discovered, his relationship as principal medical advisor becomes most important. In this role he guides the patient to the proper specialists and advises her when treatment choices are necessary. Finally, he continues follow-up care of the patient indefinitely to ensure, if possible, the long-term success of treatment.

THE BREAST MANAGEMENT TEAM: DIAGNOSIS, TREATMENT, AND REHABILITATION

Most women experience a great deal of apprehension when they are referred to a general surgeon, not realizing that a surgeon does far more than cut.

The General Surgeon's Role in a Woman's Breast Care
KENNETH J. ARNOLD, M.D.

In his practice, the general surgeon primarily treats abdominal, noncardiac chest and chest wall, peripheral vascular, body surface, and glandular surgical problems. Diseases of the breast are within this area of expertise and are an important part of a general surgeon's practice. A woman is referred to a general surgeon when the question of a difficult breast examination or a breast biopsy arises.

The surgeon ultimately decides whether a breast biopsy is to be recommended and then performs that procedure. The surgeon can and should be more than just an arbiter of operations. He should be a resource to the patient, knowledgeable about diseases of the breast and their significance, and able to answer the many questions that women have about their breasts.

For the woman with breast cancer, the general surgeon becomes her first contact about the disease. He must be able to sensitively and sensibly discuss with the woman the many controversies surrounding the issue of breast cancer and the various choices available to her. Finally, the surgeon must be able to make appropriate recommendations for treatment and then skillfully carry out the agreed on therapy, referring to other specialists as indicated and coordinating where necessary with the radiation oncologist (radiotherapist), chemotherapist (medical oncologist), and plastic surgeon.

When a woman decides to have a mastectomy to treat her breast cancer, the general surgeon will perform this surgery. Often he also will inform the woman of the option of breast reconstruction. Then if the woman is interested in this option she and her surgeon can discuss the timing for reconstruction. If she desires immediate breast restoration during the same operation as her mastectomy, the general surgeon often will refer her to a plastic surgeon, either the one on his breast management team or one with whom he has worked before.

A woman must feel comfortable with her surgeon and freely discuss any and all issues concerning her breast biopsy or cancer treatment. If she is unable to do so, she should consider seeking another surgeon who is more compatible with her needs. Among the many questions a woman might consider asking her surgeon are the following:

- How should I examine myself? What time of the month is best and what am I looking for?
- When and how often should I see a physician?
- What are my risks of breast cancer and what can I do to lessen them?
- Is mammography necessary and will it increase my risk of developing cancer?

When a biopsy is necessary, she might ask:

- Should it be done on an inpatient or outpatient basis and under local or general anesthesia?
- Where will the scar be?
- What will the aftereffects be?
- Why is this biopsy necessary? Will the whole lump be gone or just part of it? When will the result be known with certainty?
- After biopsy, how long do I have to make up my mind on treatment if it shows cancer?
- What do we do if it is cancer?
- What is removed with a mastectomy?
- What is the difference between a radical and a modified radical mastectomy?
- Do I have to have a mastectomy if I have breast cancer? Can I have any other treatment?
- If I have a mastectomy, where will the scar be and will I be able to have breast reconstruction?

For the woman who ultimately develops breast cancer or for any woman conferring with a general surgeon, no question is silly and every question that she has for her surgeon should be answered.

The Pathologist's Role in the Diagnosis and Treatment of Breast Problems
JOHN S. MEYER, M.D.

A pathologist is a medical doctor specializing in the analysis and diagnosis of disease in the laboratory. He analyzes tissues obtained from biopsies or removal of organs, performs postmortem examinations, and analyzes blood and other body fluids. He is an expert in cytology, which is the analysis of cells from tissues and fluids. In this role he will analyze Papanicolau (Pap) smears and smears of secretions from the nipple to detect malignant cells. To effectively diagnose breast cancer, the pathologist also has a thorough familiarity with the microscopic anatomy of the breast and its various diseased states.

Although the woman with a breast lump will talk to and be examined by her personal physician and surgeon, she is not likely to meet the pathologist who is responsible for diagnosing her condition if a biopsy is done. Ordinarily the specimen that the surgeon removes is sent to the laboratory, where the pathologist examines it in the light of the surgeon's findings, which are written on a form accompanying the specimen.

This examination has two steps. First is the gross examination in which the pathologist uses his naked eye to scrutinize the specimen and select portions for microscopic study. After hardening and preserving these portions in formaldehyde or some other fluid, histotechnologists prepare microscopic slides on which very thin, transparent sections of the tissues are sliced and stained to make them visible under the microscope. Next, during microscopic examination of these slides, the pathologist analyzes the types of cells present and their relationship to each other.

When analyzing a biopsy specimen, a pathologist does more than simply diagnose or rule out the presence of cancer. Breast cancer is actually not a single disease, but a classification containing many subtypes with different significance to the patient and the doctors treating her. First, the pathologist decides whether the cancer is invasive (infiltrating) or intraductal (in situ). In situ cancer, either within the breast duct or lobule, does not metastasize and is virtually 100% curable by removal of the breast. If the cancer is invasive, it is classified as to the exact type. Certain invasive cancers are slow growing and usually do not metastasize. The great majority of women with these special types of breast cancer are cured by a mastectomy and axillary lymph node dissection without any further treatment.

Most breast cancers do not belong to the special slow-growing types mentioned above. The pathologist can classify these cancers further by noting the characteristics of their cells and their patterns of growth in the breast tissues and axillary lymph nodes. If an axillary dissection has been done, he examines the lymph nodes microscopically to determine the presence or absence of carcinoma. The chances of having a recurrence of cancer or a metastasis depend strongly on the number of lymph nodes that contain cancer.

Measurement of estrogen and progesterone receptors in the cancer cells is a new method for determining the risk of cancer recurring and the subsequent need for further therapy (adjuvant chemotherapy, radiation therapy, or hormonal therapy). Carcinomas that contain large amounts of estrogen and progesterone receptors, in general, are less likely to recur or metastasize within a few years of breast removal than are carcinomas with small amounts of these receptors or no detectable receptors. Thus information about the presence or absence of estrogen and progesterone receptors is also included in the pathologist's report.

The final report issued by the pathologist diagnoses the cancer and classifies it based on the various findings previously mentioned. This report is used by the general surgeon and other members of the breast management team in assessing the woman's risks of spread or possible recurrence of her cancer and in determining the appropriate treatment for her and the need for any adjuvant therapies designed to prevent recurrence.

The identification of a breast cancer might require a woman to consult with still other members of the breast management team who will help with her treatment and rehabilitation.

The Radiation Oncologist's Role in Treating a Woman with Breast Cancer
JOHN BEDWINEK, M.D.

A radiation oncologist (also called a radiotherapist) is a doctor specializing in the treatment of cancer with irradiation, a very potent killer of cancer cells. In the past, the radiologist used irradiation to treat cancer because he had access to the use of radiation-producing machines. Today, however, with the tremendous growth in information about cancer and recent technical innovations in the application of radiation therapy, it is no longer possible for radiotherapy to be adequately delivered by a radiologist as was the case in the past. Consequently, the present day roles of the radiologist and radiation oncologist are very different. The radiologist takes x-ray pictures and interprets them; he does not treat cancer patients. The radiation oncologist, on the other hand, is a cancer expert who is directly involved in the care of cancer patients before, during, and after their treatment by irradiation. The radiation oncologist determines if and when irradiation should be used and is a part of the cancer team (surgeon, radiation oncologist, medical oncologist) that decides what is the optimum combination of the three cancer-treating modalities: surgery, irradiation, and chemotherapy. The radiation oncologist also decides how much and what type of irradiation should be used and is directly responsible for delivering the irradiation effectively and safely.

The radiation oncologist needs a broad range of training. He must be well versed in general medicine in order to be a good physician who can competently care for his patients. He also must have a thorough knowledge of all types of cancer and be knowledgeable about the capabilities, limitations, and side effects of surgery and chemotherapy. Finally, he must be well versed in nuclear physics, the effects of irradiation on human tissues, and the technical details required for precisely delivering irradiation to cancerous tissue while sparing normal tissue.

A radiation oncologist also must have compassion and sensitivity, qualities not easily taught in a formal training program. The patient who discovers that she has cancer usually has very special psychological needs, and the radiation oncologist must be sensitive to these needs and be equipped to offer the necessary support and understanding. One of the most important and helpful things that a radiation oncologist, or any doctor for that matter, should do for his patient is to offer a very clear and easily understandable explanation of the following issues:

- What is the specific kind of cancer that the patient has, and how does it grow and spread?
- What are the treatment options for this particular kind of cancer? Will it be irradiation, surgery, or chemotherapy—or a combination of these modalities?
- What is the specific purpose of each of the treatments to be used? Using an advanced breast cancer as an example, such an

explanation might go as follows: "A modified radical mastectomy, which is removal of the entire breast and lymph nodes under the arm, will be done in an attempt to remove all the cancer cells residing in the breast. Since the tumor in your breast has worked its way into the skin, a mastectomy alone might not be able to get rid of all the cancer cells; therefore, in addition to a mastectomy, we will use irradiation to kill any cancer cells that might be left behind. Also, if we find cancer in the armpit lymph nodes, there is a pretty good chance that there might be cancer cells elsewhere in your body or in the bloodstream. We will then need to give you chemotherapy, which goes all through your body, in an attempt to kill these bloodstream cancer cells."

- What are the specific side effects and potential complications of the proposed treatment and what are the chances of having any of these complications?
- What is the treatment for possible complications if they occur?
- Will the patient be able to engage in normal daily activities during the treatment. If not, what are the restrictions, and how soon can normal activity be resumed?
- Are there any alternatives to the proposed treatment and what are the chances of success and possible side effects of these alternatives?

These issues are the bare minimum that must be explained without the patient having to ask; however, there are always more questions, and the patient should be given ample opportunity to think and to ask any additional questions. The physician must make every effort to ensure that what is said is fully understood. Explanations and answers to questions should be given at least twice. It is the rare patient who can understand and fully grasp unfamiliar facts and concepts on the first explanation, particularly since she may still be in a daze from the recent discovery that she has cancer. In this regard, it is also helpful for the woman to have a close family member present when explanations are given.

Being able to explain complicated medical facts and concepts in an easily understandable fashion is, in part, a gift, but mainly it is a skill that must be acquired through patience, effort, and practice. Unfortunately, this skill is not possessed by all physicians; yet it is one of the doctor's most important responsibilities. Many in the medical profession have forgotten, or just don't know, that the origin of the title "doctor" comes from the Latin word *doceo*, which means "to teach" or "to explain." A doctor should first and foremost be a good teacher. If not, then the patient should find another doctor who is.

The Medical Oncologist's Role in Treating the Woman with Breast Cancer
GARY A. RATKIN, M.D.

A medical oncologist is a specialist in internal medicine who is knowledgeable in the management of malignant or neoplastic disease and is well versed in the common and unusual facts about each cancer that he treats.

A woman who has had initial treatment for breast cancer consults a medical oncologist when she is being considered for adjunctive therapy or when there is evidence that she has metastatic cancer. The patient usually is referred to the medical oncologist by the surgeon or her primary physician (internist, gynecologist, or general practitioner). Communication with each of these physicians is very important for the medical oncologist who will be making important recommendations to the patient with the information provided to him. The oncologist will review the original pathology report, the hormone receptor data, and any clinical data such as x-ray pictures, laboratory tests, symptoms, and physical findings. Using this information, he will advise the woman about the diagnosis, staging, and ultimate treatment of her disease.

The medical oncologist needs to have extensive knowledge and experience in handling and prescribing chemotherapy drugs. When the patient requires chemotherapy, he is the one responsible for its administration. Thus, he must know the side effects of these drugs, how to prevent these effects, or how to deal with them if they become significant complications. In particular, an in-depth knowledge of hematological (blood) problems is required, as well as broader experience in dealing with infectious diseases and lung, heart, or gastrointestinal problems. To be effective as an oncologist, the physician must be aware of the many advances involving new chemotherapy drugs, and current techniques that allow the most effective or safest administration of such agents.

The physician must know and understand the many physical and emotional problems that the cancer patient may face so that he can sensitively and humanely address her concerns and help her to cope with and understand the different aspects involved with treatment of her cancer.

Because the oncologist is knowledgeable about cancer as a disease and tries to treat the patient as an individual, he must be an expert in all of the resources available to that patient in her community. He must be aware of other physicians who are experts in their respective fields, such as radiation oncology, pathology, surgery, plastic surgery, and rehabilitation medicine. Knowledge of local nursing resources is critical, as well as knowledge of home nursing agencies, hospice programs, pharmacies that cater to the needs of cancer patients, community service organizations, dieticians, and social workers.

Finally, the medical oncologist should be a scientist, as well as a humanist. He should be able to scrutinize and criticize information 'in order to arrive at the best treatment plan. Many oncologists participate in the development of new treatment programs and help to gather and interpret information for dissemination about groups of patients. Organized hospital cancer programs, tumor registries (organized by the American College of Surgeons), and cooperative cancer study groups allow practicing physicians to continue to contribute to the development of oncology as a science of cancer management.

A woman needs to understand the reason she is seeing an oncologist. Questions about the stage of her disease and the implications it has for her life or prognosis need to be addressed to the oncologist. In addition, she should understand the goals of the suggested treatment. Further questions about the actual treatment program and how she can assess the effectiveness of treatment are very important.

Finally, she needs to understand the benefits and the potential toxicity of this treatment. The common side effects of chemotherapy must be clearly outlined and any means of preventing or ameliorating such toxic effects discussed. The woman then may have specific questions about the drug therapy as it applies to her, its timing, and its cost. She also will have questions about activities, return to work, diet, or exercise. Possible drug interactions also should be explained before chemotherapy or hormonal therapy is started. In addition, the oncologist can refer the patient to available National Institutes of Health and American Cancer Society pamphlets on chemotherapy and specific drugs.

Although a woman may have a primary physician and/or surgeon caring for her before referral to the medical oncologist, the pattern of patient follow-up may be very different after that referral. The oncologist will not only be expert in the methods for treating her cancer, but also will need to suggest means for monitoring the patient's health after her therapy is completed. The woman's health is then often monitored by the oncologist, especially during the period that active cancer treatment is underway. The exact pattern of care is established by close communication between the woman and the involved physicians.

The Plastic Surgeon's Role in the Rehabilitation of the Woman with Breast Cancer
JOHN BOSTWICK III, M.D.

Plastic surgeons treat patients with a wide range of deformities. They perform aesthetic surgical procedures to counteract the effects of the aging process and reconstructive procedures to repair major body defects, such as deformities resulting from birth defects, injuries and scars caused by accidents (including hand injuries and burns), and deformities resulting from cancer treatment.

Breast surgery is a major part of many plastic surgeons' practices. Women consult plastic surgeons for aesthetic breast operations to enlarge, reduce, or elevate their breasts and for reconstructive breast surgery to replace their missing breasts and nipple-areolae after mastectomy. Today, with recent developments in the field combined with the skills acquired from treating aesthetic breast problems, plastic surgeons are able to create aesthetically successful breast reconstructions for patients with all types of mastectomy deformities.

A woman is referred to a plastic surgeon when she is interested in the option of breast restoration. Frequently this referral is made by the general surgeon before or after a planned mastectomy. It also may be made by her family physician or by another member of the breast management team, of which the plastic surgeon is a part. Many women come to the plastic surgeon after referral by other women who have been treated by him for similar problems.

When a woman consults with a plastic surgeon about breast reconstruction, he must consider her psychological state, the stage of her disease, and her need for additional therapy. Management of her tumor is a primary concern, and he will confer with the general surgeon and other members of the team to determine the best care for each woman and the best timing for her reconstruction. When immediate reconstruction is planned, he works closely with the general surgeon to coordinate the mastectomy and reconstruction for the patient.

The plastic surgeon is also aware of the ongoing concerns that a woman has about her cancer and must deal with her in a humane and sensitive fashion. A woman who is considering breast reconstruction has had to cope with the reality of breast cancer, as well as with the loss of her breast. The emotional trauma that she has experienced should never be overlooked by the plastic surgeon in his dealings with her. He needs to provide support and understanding for the special problems and fears that she, as a cancer patient, is confronting.

The plastic surgeon also must be aware of some of the conflicts faced by the woman who inquires about reconstructive breast surgery. Although a woman wants to have her breast restored, she also may fear that reconstructive surgery will cause a recurrence of her cancer. The plastic surgeon needs to be sensitive to this fear and discuss it with his prospective patient. She also may worry that this elective surgery will be misconstrued as mere vanity on her part. The plastic surgeon's role is to reassure her that breast reconstruction is not a cosmetic procedure, but is a beneficial part of her total rehabilitation program.

Counseling patients is an important part of the plastic surgeon's practice, and this activity takes place before breast reconstruction and sometimes before mastectomy. Consultations should be conducted in a private, quiet atmosphere to enable a woman to feel comfortable and free to speak frankly.

As a counselor, one of the plastic surgeon's chief obligations is to be a good listener. If he does all of the talking, he will never really know what the woman's expectations are for treatment. He should ask open-ended questions that allow her to communicate her feelings and desires. He needs to understand what a woman expects, so that he can design an operation to most nearly produce her desired result. If her expectations cannot be met, he needs to explain the limitations of what surgery can accomplish.

The patient's medical history and the status and treatment of her breast cancer provide important information needed by a plastic surgeon in formulating a plan for breast reconstruction. He also will perform a physical examination to assess the options for reconstruction. These options then can be discussed with the woman. In this discussion, the pros and cons, expected results, and risks of each approach should be addressed. Breast reconstruction is a very personal procedure and the woman should understand that no one surgical technique is appropriate for all patients. An operative plan is designed with an individual woman's specific needs in mind.

After these explanations, the plastic surgeon can formulate an operative plan that attempts to incorporate his patient's desires and expectations. He should not assume, however, that a woman will naturally understand the details of her proposed surgery and should carefully review this plan with her.

The actual breast reconstruction is carried out by the plastic surgeon according to the preoperative plan that he and the patient have discussed and agreed on. After reconstruction, the woman returns to the plastic surgeon for periodic evaluations. In his patient follow-up, the plastic surgeon will continue to encourage his patient and to contribute to her rehabilitation from breast cancer. (For further information on selecting and communicating with a plastic surgeon, see Chapter 9.)

THE TEAM EFFORT

Many specialists become involved in the care of the woman with breast cancer. Some are her primary care doctors whom she has known and visited for years. She feels comfortable with them and trusts their judgment. Others, however, are specialists whom she sees for the first time on referral for treatment of her life-threatening illness. The thought of seeing strange doctors is often intimidating to an already stressed woman. Knowledge of what these doctors do and the positive benefit they can provide for the woman with breast cancer might alleviate some of her fears of this experience and help her to feel less terrified and alone. This chapter has been designed to provide this information for women and to demonstrate how the team functions at its best and how individual doctors, regardless of specialty, can deal with their patients with caring and sensitivity.

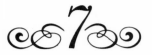

WHY WOMEN SEEK BREAST RECONSTRUCTION

I was planting seedlings one day and my prosthesis fell out while I was bending over. Crying, I picked it up out of the muddy water. I called a plastic surgeon that same day.

I ached to once again be able to put on a beautiful nightgown and fill it all out. I wanted to shop for pretty things and feel feminine and sexy again.

I was only 17, an oddity for breast cancer patients. I had a long life to live, and I wanted to live it whole.

THIS CHAPTER OPENS with just three of the many different responses that we received when we surveyed and interviewed women who had undergone breast reconstruction. Their motives for seeking reconstructive surgery were diverse, but all were touching manifestations of the sense of personal loss that these women had experienced after their mastectomies. For some women the mastectomy has been an experience that left them feeling "ugly" and "lopsided." Reconstruction therefore represented a means of regaining beauty and wholeness, harmony of body. For these women femininity was a core issue, and they felt that their "mastectomy appearance" deprived them of feeling fully female. They loathed the very sight of their bodies and found simple bathing to be repugnant. The mirror had become a fearsome presence in their homes. Furthermore, they avoided any situation in which they might have to disrobe in front of others — dressing rooms, locker rooms, the beach. For a good number of these women, dressing and undressing had become a strictly private act, conducted in closed bedrooms, closets, or bathrooms, until they had their breasts rebuilt and no longer felt the need to hide their bodies.

As one woman explained, "I am again a woman in my own mind. I don't look down anymore and cringe. I just know that something is there, and it has changed my whole life." Clearly an improved self-image was one of the chief reasons for desiring breast reconstruction expressed by all of the women we surveyed. This elective plastic surgery allowed them to feel more relaxed and more positive about the future.

Relatively few of the women in our survey sought breast reconstruction because it would improve the quality of their sex lives or help to save their marriages or relationships. Motivation for reconstructive surgery was usually self-inspired. The ability to contribute to and feel good in a relationship, however, was often helped when a woman had breast reconstruction. By making her feel better about herself, this operation allowed her to relate to others, especially loved ones, with increased confidence and self-assurance.

The search for restitution and return to wholeness was a strong motivating factor for all of the women we interviewed and this reason also pervaded all of the answers to our questionnaire. Even when the results of reconstruction were not perfect, the woman's dissatisfaction seemed to be minimal because the breast was now a part of her body and could again be incorporated into her self-image. As one woman said, "The reconstruction is not like a normal breast; there are some problems. It is too hard and it shifts around, but I wouldn't go back to the way I was for anything. I love my new breast, hardness and all. I am not embarrassed to undress in front of someone now. I don't feel like a freak anymore. I feel like a sexual person again. I am whole again."

Elimination of the need for an external prosthesis was another important reason why many women elected to have reconstructive surgery. Women seemed to feel constantly aware of the presence of a false breast, worrying that it would become dislodged and the lopsided chest would be exposed. In their attempts to hide their deformity some women even resorted to using surgical tape to solidly fix their false breasts to their chests.

Other women, who were large breasted, objected to the size and weight of the prosthesis necessary for symmetry with their large breast. For these women, the weight of the prosthesis created a physical imbalance and they felt as if they were being pulled to one side. Furthermore, the heavier the prosthesis, the greater its tendency to pull away from the woman's body, resulting in her effort to counterbalance this force by holding herself very straight. Some women actually said that they developed back problems and were unable to function without pain and disability. One woman, whose remaining breast was a bra size 41, had to be helped up from bed in the morning, because the strain on her back had become so severe and debilitating.

The fit and coverage of the prosthesis was another area of concern and displeasure for women. Women with radical mastectomies consistently stated that the external prosthesis did not provide adequate coverage for their deformities. Their prostheses served primarily for filling out the form of their missing breasts; they did nothing to restore the anterior fold of the axilla or fill the upper chest area just under the collarbone.

Because a woman's prosthesis is fitted to provide breast symmetry when she is upright, with her arms at her side, it does not move with her and is often unsuitable for the athletic woman who actively participates in sports. Accounts of prostheses that fell out on the tennis courts or slipped over to a woman's armpit during running or aerobic exercise were prevalent in our interviews and the source of much embarrassment to the women involved. With strenuous activity, this artificial breast was easily displaced or dislodged and could even float out of a bathing suit during swimming. It also could prevent the escape of heat from a woman's chest and cause skin irritation and skin rashes. Thus, for practical reasons of movement and comfort, many women felt that an external prosthesis was a nuisance and an inconvenience. "My prosthesis gets in my way. It interferes when I clean, exercise, or bend over." As one woman explained, "Prosthetic devices may be great in the beginning, but they are not totally comfortable. With breast reconstruction, one can feel whole again with no shifting of the prosthesis." The freedom afforded by reconstruction was emphasized by another woman who complained, "I enjoy being active; I am a swimmer and a golfer. My first prosthesis was large to match the existing breast, and it was cumbersome and floated when I dived."

For many women, one of the real bonuses of breast reconstruction was the increased variety of style and cut it allowed them in clothing. Reconstruction eliminated their need "to shop for clothes with higher necklines and specially designed swimwear." They now gained pleasure from the very act of shopping for clothing and once again felt excited about the possibility of purchasing lacy lingerie, pretty bras, and attractive blouses. Proud of their newfound ability to display a cleavage if they desired, they were also secure in the knowledge that when they were dressed there was absolutely no way that anyone could ever tell that their breasts had been reconstructed.

Before they had breast reconstruction, none of these women regarded their prosthesis as a part of them or as a new breast. It seems never to have been incorporated into their body image, but instead was regarded as a necessity, a symbol of something *missing* and a constant reminder of the real breast. These women repeatedly emphasized their need to feel less obsessed with the cancer experience and a desire to rid themselves of their sense of deformity, which had resulted from having a mastectomy. Some felt that breast reconstruction relieved them of a cancer "stigma."

Interesting also was the reaction of a group of older women we surveyed. These individuals, in their late sixties and seventies, did not have reconstructive surgery because it was not a viable alternative when they had their mastectomies. They now felt that they were too old to bother with additional surgery. These women readily agreed, however, that if their daughters were to develop breast cancer and require mastectomies (and their daughters had an increased risk) they would urge their children to have their breasts restored. For these women, breast reconstruction represented an exciting option and they felt that it would be "wonderful to have two breasts again."

In further examining motivations for seeking breast reconstruction, we noticed a definite correlation between the age and marital status of a woman and her corresponding interest in reconstructive breast surgery.

Today, breast cancer is occurring with increasing frequency in young women. Moreover, breast cancer occurs with greater frequency in women who have never had children. Concomitantly, there are more childless women who are single than married. A mastectomy and the resultant deformity pose a number of especially uncomfortable and difficult questions for single women in the early stages of an intimate relationship.

How does one explain a missing breast to a potential lover? Some of the questions raised by women facing this situation follow:

- Do I tell my date I had a mastectomy?
- What is the right timing for this disclosure? Before or after discovery?
- Do I keep my body covered while we are having sex?
- Will I continue to be seen as desirable after I admit to a deformity?

- Can I feel sexy and good about myself with a deformity? Or is it easier to avoid sexual situations?

Many woman take up the last option—preferring to steer clear of relationships that might lead to sexual intimacy. As one woman expressed it, "I could not face my life with just one breast. I was 42 years old and single when I had my mastectomy. I buried my sexuality for 13 months until I had the reconstruction."

Just as single and divorced women interested in meeting men and beginning new relationships often cite reconstruction as an attractive option, some widows reported feeling that breast surgery might be one step in a personal program of "starting over." Although many women who have had mastectomies after age 65 decide not to have additional elective surgery, age alone has no relationship to how women feel about themselves. Women at any age feel the sense of loss when they have a mastectomy. They still desire to return to wholeness. Many of the breast reconstruction patients we interviewed were over 50, and they felt that this surgery had renewed and invigorated them. In fact, some of the happiest and most satisfied women who have had breast reconstruction have been in these older age groups.

For many women, reconstruction is a symbol that they are completing the treatment and rehabilitation phase of their lives and are ready to get back to living. When the surgeon recommends reconstruction, he is saying that he feels good about the woman's chances for survival. In these cases, reconstruction represents a positive and reassuring statement from the general surgeon.

Reasons women seek reconstruction are as varied and individual as are the women themselves. Some women focus on the practical considerations of comfort and convenience, whereas others have psychological and aesthetic concerns; reconstruction bolsters their sense of femininity, self-confidence, and sexual attractiveness. Still other women seek peace of mind about the cancer experience, a realignment of their body image, and a return to wholeness. No one answer is better or more important than any other. The fact remains that after a woman's breast has been removed, a deformity exists and many women feel a deep sense of loss. The desire for restitution is a healthy reaction to this problem. It helps a woman to reconfirm her body image and bring her self-awareness back into harmony. For those women who feel the need to rebuild their bodies and replace their missing breast or breasts, reconstruction offers a positive source of hope for the future.

QUESTIONS FREQUENTLY ASKED ABOUT BREAST RECONSTRUCTION

BREAST RECONSTRUCTION is a frequently misunderstood form of surgery. Although many women desire the operation, some hesitate to request it, fearing that it is not appropriate for them. Some worry that reconstruction can cause cancer or mask a recurrence. Others have anxieties about the appearance of the new breast, the prominence of scars, or the development of further complications. Still others are concerned about the costs and the correct timing for surgery.

Some queries are so frequently posed to the doctor half of our writing team that we have prepared the following list of questions and answers to serve as a primer.

Who is a candidate for breast restoration?

Today most mastectomy patients can have their breasts rebuilt; age is not a factor in determining a woman's suitability nor is her type of mastectomy or the placement of her mastectomy scar. Women who have had radical mastectomies (removing the breast and chest wall muscles) or modified radical mastectomies (the breast removed but chest wall muscles intact) can now have satisfactory breast reconstructions. It does not matter how much time has elapsed since a woman's original cancer surgery because there is no statute of limitations for reconstruction and no disadvantage to waiting. Women have had successful reconstructive breast surgery as long as 15 to 20 years later.

How does a person's age affect the success of reconstructive surgery? Are you ever too old?

A woman's age is not as important a factor in determining the ultimate success of her breast reconstruction as is her emotional motivation for the operation and her general health. Many women in their seventies have had successful reconstructive breast surgery and are very pleased with the results of this operation. A woman is never too old if she is in good health and the type of reconstruction selected is compatible with her general physical condition.

Does the size and extent of a woman's cancer have any influence on whether she should have her breast reconstructed?

Women with small tumors have the best prognosis for survival and breast reconstruction is most frequently performed on these women. Women with large tumors that have spread to the lymph nodes also may have their breasts restored, but the timing of their operation is influenced by the type of adjunctive treatment they require.

Are women with advanced disease eligible for this operation?

Occasionally, a woman whose breast cancer has spread throughout her system requests this surgery. When this happens, the surgeon must reconcile the woman's present health status with her desire for a better life. Should he operate on a woman whose prognosis is poor and who may not live to enjoy her restored breast? Is this surgery worth the time, pain, and money it will cost when the potential time for enjoyment may be limited? For this woman, reconstruction must be discussed and performed in the context of improving the quality of her remaining life. Many women desire this procedure despite the presence of systemic disease. As one woman explained, "Even if I die tomorrow, it was worth it. I want to go out just like I came in." If the woman's motivation is strong and if she is fully informed about this surgery, then her psychological and emotional needs must be an important consideration in a decision for reconstruction. Women with advanced disease can have reconstructive surgery and some surgeons feel that these women are among their most satisfied patients. This decision for breast reconstruction cannot be made in isolation and requires consultation and follow-up with the breast management team. The final decision must be made by a well-informed patient.

Are there some women who are not suitable for breast reconstruction?

Yes, some women should not have breast reconstruction if their emotional state or personal circumstances indicate that a major operation and recuperation could be too much for them to effectively cope with.

Women in poor general health also may not be suitable for this operation. For example, if a woman has advanced diabetes mellitus, a recent stroke or heart attack, or severe chronic lung disease, she should not be considered for this procedure.

Will breast reconstruction cause cancer?

There is no evidence of any kind that breast reconstruction causes cancer to grow or makes it recur.

Will the reconstruction and the breast implant hide the recurrence of cancer or prevent the detection of a new cancer?

Local recurrence of breast cancer usually occurs in the mastectomy scar or the skin flaps. There is little difficulty in detecting an early local recurrence because the breast implant is beneath the skin and often even beneath the chest wall muscle.

Will a woman be able to feel tumors as easily after reconstruction?

After reconstruction with an implant beneath the muscle layer or with the back (latissimus dorsi) flap, the skin and scar are actually pushed forward, and new tumors or local recurrences usually can be easily felt. Detection of tumors may be somewhat more difficult when a woman's breast has been reconstructed with the lower abdominal (rectus abdominis) flap. Because this tissue is moved a long way, it sometimes develops firm, thickened areas that may be confused with a local recurrence.

What is the best placement of a mastectomy scar for the woman who desires breast reconstruction?

The best placement for this scar is in an oblique position, extending from the lower axilla to the inner lower breast area. This scar is easily covered by a brassiere, and frequently a portion of the scar can be reopened and the implant placed through it to avoid creating a new incision and thus a new scar. Sometimes, however, the primary cancer is located in an area of the breast that makes it impossible for the surgeon to leave an oblique scar.

What happens if the mastectomy scar is in a bad position?

Breast reconstruction can be done with a mastectomy scar in any position. The scar position cannot be changed, but the reconstructive implant can be positioned through this scar and the scar revised to provide the best possible appearance.

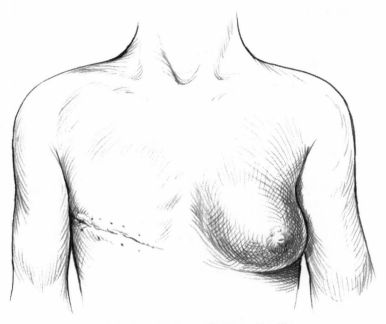

Mastectomy Scar in Oblique Position

How much tissue has to be left to allow for breast reconstruction?

A woman's breast can be reconstructed regardless of the amount of tissue remaining after the mastectomy. When the pectoralis major muscle and sufficient skin remain, a simple reconstruction with an implant or an expander followed by an implant can be done. When much of the skin or pectoralis major muscle is missing, a flap, either from the back or lower abdomen, is usually necessary.

What can be reconstructed? Can large deformities and chest hollowness be filled in?

Breast reconstruction can now give predictably good restoration of the breast shape, contour, and size. It often improves (but does not remove) scars, skin grafts, or radiation damaged skin. The upper chest and axillary deformity after a radical mastectomy can be filled in and corrected. The infraclavicular area can be rebuilt, and the missing anterior axillary fold can be recreated. Restoration of these areas, however, requires the use of additional donor tissue from the back or lower abdomen, and the subsequent creation of new scars in these areas.

Will an implant or the woman's own tissues be better for reconstruction?

This is difficult to answer because the specific method of reconstruction must be determined on an individual basis. This topic is discussed fully in Chapter 10.

Breasts reconstructed with implants can look and feel quite natural. Sometimes, however, thick fibrous tissue develops around these implants, causing them to feel firm and reducing the attractiveness of the breast. Placement of the implant under the muscle usually helps to minimize any potential hardening.

Reconstruction with a woman's own tissue avoids the use of a foreign implant material and produces a soft, natural reconstructed breast that will not become firm. She pays a price for these advantages, however. When the lower abdominal tissue is shifted to a woman's breast area, the surgeon must create additional scars on the breast and lower abdomen. This is the most complicated procedure for breast reconstruction and is associated with more pain, a longer recovery, and more postoperative complications.

What types of implants are used for breast reconstruction?

A silicone implant is often inserted under a woman's skin or muscle to create a breast mound during breast reconstruction. Basically two different types of implants are available: those that contain a silicone gel or those that can be inflated with saline (salt water). All of these implants use a silicone layer as the outer material in contact with the body tissues. A silicone gel implant with an outer layer of polyurethane foam is sometimes used in breast reconstruction to protect against hardening of the implant. An implant with a double-layered envelope, called a double-lumen implant, is also available. This implant combines features from the two different types to include an inner envelope containing silicone gel and an outer envelope that can be inflated with a small volume of saline.

Is it necessary for the woman's normal breast to be modified to match the new one?

Many times a good match can be achieved with a simple implant placement and without touching a woman's normal breast. Sometimes, to avoid altering the opposite breast, it may be necessary to reconstruct the missing breast with a flap procedure. When the normal breast is very large and sagging or flat and small, the surgeon may not be able to match it and some modification might be required. (See Chapters 11 and 12 for additional information on this subject.)

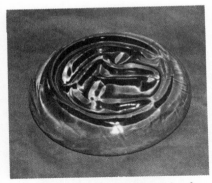

Silicone Gel-filled Implant

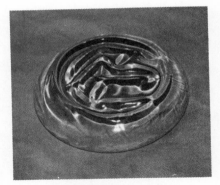

Saline-filled Implant

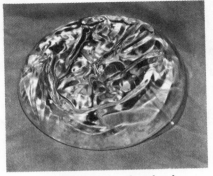

Double-Lumen Implant

Can the missing nipple be reconstructed?

Yes. Both the central projecting nipple and the darker surrounding areola can be reconstructed, and this procedure is usually done as a second operation. (See Chapter 13 for more detailed information.)

What type of new scars are created by reconstruction?

Reconstruction using the existing tissues or by expanding the existing tissues requires only the mastectomy scar, and no new scar is necessary. This is the most frequently used approach. Sometimes, if new skin must be added to the reconstructed breast, additional scars are necessary to inset this skin into the breast. New scars on the breast usually extend along the lower breast crease and either up to the old scar or up to the nipple level.

Whenever new tissue is added, scars are the necessary result of obtaining this tissue. Common donor sites are the back, side, and abdomen. Scars from the back are either across the back or under the arm. The abdominal scar is usually across the lower abdomen just above the pubic hair line.

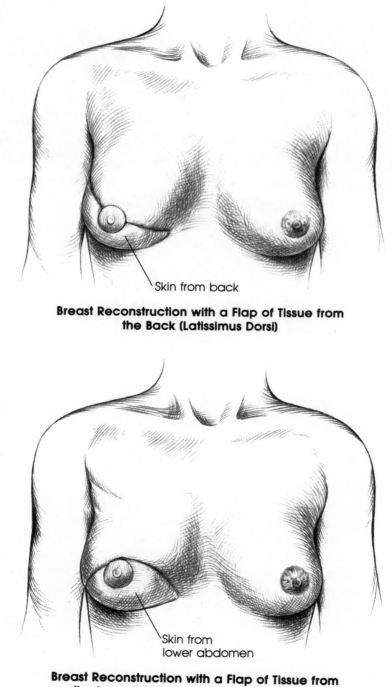

Skin from back

**Breast Reconstruction with a Flap of Tissue from
the Back (Latissimus Dorsi)**

Skin from
lower abdomen

**Breast Reconstruction with a Flap of Tissue from
the Lower Abdomen (Rectus Abdominis)**

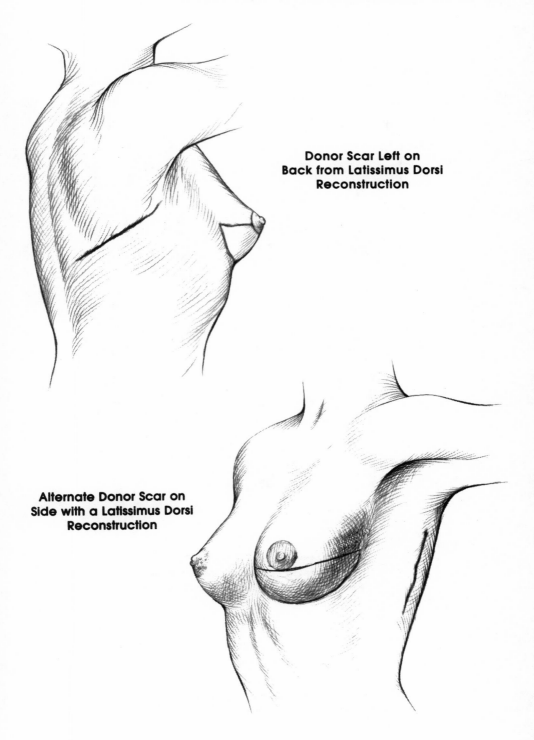

**Donor Scar Left on
Back from Latissimus Dorsi
Reconstruction**

**Alternate Donor Scar on
Side with a Latissimus Dorsi
Reconstruction**

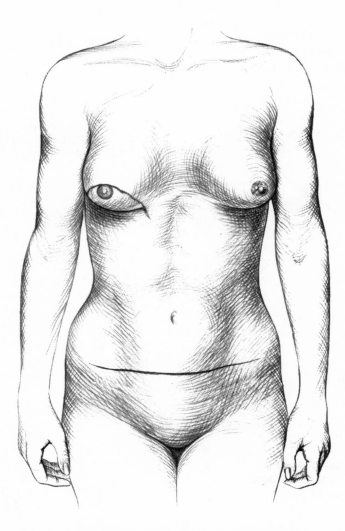

**Donor Scar on Lower Abdomen from
Rectus Abdominis Reconstruction**

Can the plastic surgeon totally remove the mastectomy scar when he restores the new breast?

The scars from the mastectomy cannot be removed, although they sometimes can be reduced or made less obvious by a plastic surgical procedure called *scar revision*. A scar line will always be present where the original cancer surgery was performed. Initially the scar will be red and raised, a condition that will persist for several months after the operation. This redness (indicative of increased blood flow from the healing process) and thickness will subside over the next 1 to 2 years as the scars improve in appearance and become less obvious. Scars in fair-skinned women tend to remain red for a longer period of time. It takes less time for the scars of older women to fade. Some women heal with thick scars, and this tendency is obvious from the appearance of the mastectomy scar, as well as any other scars that they may have.

Can another person tell, if he or she doesn't already know, if a woman has had breast reconstruction?

A woman who has had breast reconstruction can expect to dress normally without anyone realizing that her breast has been rebuilt. Unless she is naked, her scars will not be noticeable to anyone, and her clothed breasts will appear the same as any other woman's.

If a woman has reconstruction, will she be able to wear V necklines and ordinary clothing without high necks?

A woman who has had a modified radical mastectomy with a scar that falls under her brassiere will be able to wear V necklines again. If she has had a radical mastectomy, with removal of the pectoralis major muscle, reconstruction (which requires flap tissue) can still permit her to wear V-neck clothing unless the mastectomy scar extends into this central area of the chest and she doesn't want it to show.

Sports clothes also can be worn, but sometimes the style might have to accommodate any unusually positioned mastectomy scar or a donor flap scar on her back, underarm, or lower abdomen.

If a person gains or loses a considerable amount of weight, how will that weight change affect the results of breast reconstruction?

For some women, general weight losses or gains are reflected in their breasts; in others they are not. After an implant reconstruction, a major weight change will probably produce a change in the normal breast and result in the development of breast asymmetry. This asymmetry may require an implant change (an outpatient procedure.)

Reconstructions with patients' own lower abdominal tissues usually remain symmetrical under these circumstances because of the major fatty components of both the normal and reconstructed breasts.

How do the results of breast reconstruction compare with a woman's expectations for this surgery? Do her breasts look and feel normal?

It is important for a woman to carefully define her expectations before she has this operation to make sure that the plastic surgeon knows what she wants and can tell her if it is possible. Breast reconstruction can fill in and rebuild the deformities resulting from her mastectomy. A woman may be disappointed, however, if she expects her new breast to be the same as the one it is meant to replace. Her new breast will often be harder and more rounded than her remaining one is. It will not move as naturally with changes in position or posture. This firmness is often associated with the use of silicone implants. A more normal breast "feel" and flow can sometimes be obtained by using the patient's own tissue from the lower abdomen.

Because sensation or feeling in the chest wall area is lost during the mastectomy, the reconstructed breast is usually numb or at least has less sensation than the normal side. The underarm is also numb and feels strange to touch. Some women say that shaving their underarms becomes a rather uncomfortable experience. Additional numbness usually exists on the underside of the upper arm.

A woman also will be disillusioned if she desires this surgery to remedy preexisting personal problems, repair a faltering relationship, or please another individual. To be worthwhile, a woman's rebuilt chest must satisfy her personal, but reasonable, expectations.

What are the psychological benefits from breast reconstruction?

Each woman benefits from breast reconstruction in her own personal and individual manner. Many women who have had their breasts rebuilt have said that this operation made them "feel better about themselves, normal or whole again." Some women indicated that it relieved them of a constant reminder of the cancer and the mastectomy. Other women were pleased at the freedom it afforded them without the need for an external prosthesis. (See Chapters 7, 14, and 15 for more information.)

How will a woman's breast reconstruction affect her relationship with her husband, family, friends, or loved ones?

A breast reconstruction usually does not change interpersonal relationships. It can, however, give the woman a boost in self-esteem, improve her feelings about herself, and therefore permit her to more thoroughly enjoy the normal relationships and activities of her life.

Is there any depression after this operation?

Some women experience a limited but normal period of depression after breast reconstruction. The operation, general anesthesia, postoperative pain, and medications may combine to produce these feelings. Because this operation represents a major step for a woman, there is an emotional buildup to prepare for it, as well as heightened expectations of a lovely result. Therefore, a woman may be let down once the operation is over because the final result will not be obvious in the postoperative period. Instead, her breast may look bruised and possibly flat, far removed from the result she expected. This depression usually subsides in a few days as the patient recovers and the appearance of her breast improves.

What aftereffects and adjustments should a woman expect after breast reconstruction? What is the anticipated pain and recovery time?

After breast reconstruction, a woman will experience pain in her chest area, as well as in any donor sites where additional tissue was taken to build her new breast. The degree of pain and length of the recuperative period will vary with the individual patient, the extent of her defect, and the operative procedure chosen. (Specific information on these matters is provided in great detail in Chapter 10.)

Her breast may appear smaller than expected and bruised. It may not be completely symmetrical with the opposite breast. With time some asymmetries will lessen or if they persist, they usually can be adjusted a few months later during a second procedure and at the time of the nipple-areola reconstruction.

When an expander is used, the reconstructed breast will look smaller at first. It will be enlarged during several postoperative visits when additional saline is added to the expander.

What are possible complications from breast reconstruction? When do they occur and why?

Complications of breast reconstruction appear either immediately after the operation or develop later. The type and degree of complications occurring are related to the method of reconstruction used.

When an implant or expander is used to reconstruct the breast with the existing tissues, a blood collection (hematoma) can develop around the implant; this problem usually requires drainage, often in an operating room. When the skin is thin or irradiated, actual exposure of the implant can occur because of the poor cover. Infection also may occur.

Complications are more possible after flap reconstructions. Hematoma may occur in both the site of the reconstruction or in the donor sites. If the flap tissue that is moved does not have an adequate blood supply, a portion or occasionally the entire flap may be lost.

Capsular contracture is the most frequent late problem; this topic is addressed in the next discussion.

What is capsular contracture and what causes it?

A capsular contracture is a firm, fibrous scar that forms around a breast implant; the contracture is caused by a reaction of the body to the implant. This is a characteristic response of the body to protect itself from any unnatural, foreign substance. This scar tissue may become hard, thick, and constrict the implant, thus producing a rounded, spherical appearance to the breast. We do not know what causes this reaction to the implant. When the contracture is mild, no treatment is necessary. More significant contractures may require an operation to release the scar. During this secondary operation the surgeon may reposition the implant under the pectoralis major muscle; if it previously was placed over the muscle, he may select a different implant, or he may add a small amount of saline. Some women decide to have these firm breasts managed by removing the implant and scar tissue and replacing it with fatty flap tissue from the lower abdomen.

Does the body ever reject any part used in reconstruction?

Silicone is one of the most nonreactive and inert of the implantable materials. The body does not actually "reject" this material. It can, however, respond to it by creating a layer of scar tissue that, when thickened, is identified as a capsular contracture. When this contracture develops beneath thinned breast skin, it can produce a hole in the skin, and the exposed implant may have to be removed.

When the reconstruction is done with the patient's own flap tissue, rejection is not expected. Complications such as decreased blood supply of the transferred tissue and drainage can be interpreted by some as a rejection phenomenon, when in fact they are not.

Do flaps used in breast reconstruction ever die or fail? If so, what can be done to complete the reconstruction?

Flaps are an essential component of some reconstructions. A flap is a portion of tissue that is moved from one area of the body to another. For the flap to be successful, a plentiful blood supply must remain in the transferred tissue. If this blood supply is marginal or partially insufficient, a portion of the flap can die; this portion of the flap is therefore lost as a source of tissue for reconstruction.

Usually reconstruction can be completed even with partial flap loss. Rarely is the entire blood supply to the flap impaired and the entire flap lost. Potential flap loss usually can be identified during the operation and appropriate measures taken by the surgeon to avoid this problem. Certain general health conditions of the woman can impair blood supply to flaps and result in flap loss; for instance, if a woman has diabetes, has received radiation to the vessels of her flap, or is a cigarette smoker, she may have reduced blood flow.

Can a woman die from breast reconstruction?

The risks to life from breast reconstruction are very low. One obvious risk is from anesthesia; today, however, administration of anesthetics is safe in the hands of well-trained anesthesiologists. Reconstruction with implants is also safe. Flap reconstructions, especially with the lower abdominal flap, carry some risks because of the length of these operations and the risk of blood loss and the development of blood clots in the woman's legs.

How many operations are needed for breast reconstruction?

Aesthetically acceptable reconstructions usually can be completed in two operations. The first operation includes the reconstruction of the chest wall and breast mound and adjustments of the remaining breast (if indicated). A possible operation on the other breast would include enlargement, reduction, or uplifting to allow both breasts to eventually be more nearly the same size and position (Chapter 11). The second procedure is less extensive and includes nipple-areola reconstruction (Chapter 13) and any additional operations that im-prove breast symmetry. One-stage procedures (building both the breast and nipple-areola in one operation) have a higher incidence of malposition of the nipple-areola and breast asymmetries; these problems can be avoided with a two-stage procedure.

What are the timing options for breast reconstruction?

Once a woman has decided that she wants breast reconstruction, timing is important. When should this elective surgery be per-formed? For some women, the decision is made by circumstance, be-cause they are unaware that reconstruction is possible until long after the mastectomy has been performed. Today, however, with in-creased emphasis on informed consent, many women learn of the option of reconstruction from their general surgeons before they have their mastectomies and have the opportunity to contact a plas-tic surgeon or several (for different opinions) to discuss reconstruc-tive surgery and the correct timing for this procedure.

Reconstruction can be performed immediately at the same time as the mastectomy or during the same hospital stay, or it can be per-formed on a delayed basis, a few days, several months, or many years after the initial mastectomy.

What are the advantages of immediate reconstruction?

Immediate reconstruction, or reconstructive surgery performed at the same time as the mastectomy, has a definite psychological ap-peal for many women. The prospect of having a life-threatening breast cancer and simultaneously facing the loss of a breast is devas-tating to most women. Some women even delay medical help and re-fuse a mastectomy because they fear losing a breast. Some women will not consider a mastectomy unless they can have immediate breast reconstruction. Others decide to have a lumpectomy and ra-diation therapy.

Recent studies by Schain (1983), Noone et al. (1982), and Dow-den (1979) reveal that immediate reconstruction has positive psy-chological benefits for women who wish to rid themselves of their preoccupation with cancer and breast loss. Furthermore, these women are, for the most part, satisfied with the results of their im-mediate surgery. The Schain study indicates that women having im-mediate breast reconstruction express less overall psychological trauma associated with their mastectomies and recall less intensely the pain of their initial cancer surgery. They incorporate their new breasts more quickly into a redefined body image and exhibit a lower level of distress, probably because they awaken from the mastectomy with a breast contour intact and thus do not experience the degree of self-consciousness that accompanies breast amputation. They also do not feel the anxiety associated with camouflaging the defect or having the external prosthesis become dislodged. These women are not any more or less appreciative of what has been done for them, and many are particularly grateful that they did not have to live without their breast or breasts for any period of time.

Other advantages to recommend an immediate procedure include the reduced cost of having reconstruction performed in one hospitalization, with only one anesthesia and one operation.

What are the disadvantages of an immediate procedure?

Some plastic surgeons believe the results they achieve with immediate reconstruction are not as good for many women as those they attain with delayed reconstruction. Symmetry is sometimes difficult to produce in one operation, and the reconstructed breast usually is not as natural in appearance as a breast created with a delayed procedure. When the nipple-areola is replaced at the time of the mastectomy, its ideal position also may be hard to determine. Therefore, immediate reconstruction usually does not include a nipple-areola; this is delayed until a second operation. Furthermore, most surgeons do not want to operate on the remaining breast at the time of the mastectomy.

There is also a higher complication rate from skin loss, hematoma, and infection with immediate reconstruction. The mastectomy wound, fluid accumulation (seroma), and low-grade infections add to the potential for fibrous formation around the implant, possibly resulting in capsular contracture or hardening of the reconstructed breast.

Some plastic surgeons fear that a less than perfect reconstruction could cause further psychological distress for an already stressed patient. Since the patient has not seen the mastectomy deformity, she can only compare the reconstruction with her normal breast. Many plastic surgeons and women who have had a delayed reconstruction feel that the mastectomy experience is traumatic enough without adding a reconstruction to it. Since reconstruction is for a lifetime, the woman should have the best possible result, which additional time may help the surgeon to achieve.

Close teamwork between the general surgeon and the plastic surgeon is required for this surgical approach. The general surgeon should be supportive of the decision for immediate breast reconstruction, and he must work with the plastic surgeon to plan and carry out this operation.

There are obvious benefits and risks to be considered in immediate reconstruction. They are summarized as follows:

Benefits	Risks
Immediate replacement of breast	Result may not be as aesthetic as a delayed reconstruction
Psychological satisfaction and relief	Allows no time for physicians to assess the needs for additional therapy that may be required
Avoidance of trauma attending the mastectomy experience	
Reduced cost and hospitalization time	Higher complication rate and longer operative time

Who are suitable candidates for immediate reconstruction?

The women most suitable for immediate reconstruction have small tumors (about 1 inch in diameter or less) and no involved axillary lymph nodes (indicating less likelihood that the cancer has spread beyond their breast tissue). To achieve the best possible aesthetic result, the plastic surgeon prefers immediate surgery for women with small breasts because it is easier to match the remaining breast. Symmetry also is facilitated for women who are having both breasts removed (because there is a better chance for achieving symmetry).

What are the advantages of delayed reconstruction?

Delayed reconstruction can be performed from a few days to years after the mastectomy. For patients with stage I disease who do not require chemotherapy or radiation therapy, many plastic surgeons prefer to reconstruct these women's breasts 3 to 6 months after their mastectomies.

Delayed surgery affords the woman time to cope with her initial cancer. In recent interviews with seven women who had delayed reconstruction, these women were asked if they would have preferred to have had their reconstruction done immediately. Although two admitted that they could have had the procedure earlier than they did (after 11- and 3-year delays), they all felt that a waiting period was necessary to allow them to "cope with their cancer, get their emotional lives in order, and separate the negative cancer experience from the very positive reconstruction." In addition, these patients also felt that by delaying their surgery they had more time to investigate their reconstructive surgery and thus had more realistic expectations about what reconstructive surgery could provide.

By delaying her reconstructive surgery, a woman has time to fully evaluate her decision to have her breast rebuilt; some women change their minds after a waiting period and decide not to pursue this option. This time also allows a woman to recover from any additional therapy that might be required and to fully explore the topic of reconstruction, find the right plastic surgeon, get to know him, and decide on the correct reconstructive approach.

For the plastic surgeon, delay offers the psychological benefit of a patient committed to this procedure. In addition, the plastic surgeon and general surgeon often desire, for health considerations, to know the full extent of the patient's disease and to help her understand the extent of her cancer and the anticipated treatment before she embarks on further surgery.

Aesthetically, the chances of an improved result are better with delayed reconstruction than with immediate reconstruction, although the results obtained with immediate reconstruction have improved over the years. Delayed reconstruction allows the breast tissues time to heal, soften, and settle. The surgeon can then plan his surgery more effectively to achieve breast symmetry and accurate placement of the nipple-areola (if it is to be reconstructed). With delayed reconstruction, a woman is more likely to get a result that truly meets her aesthetic and personal expectations. The plastic surgeon can feel in control of the variables of the reconstruction better than when a new operation is initiated at the end of a mastectomy operation.

What are the disadvantages of a delayed procedure?

One of the primary disadvantages of a delayed procedure is the period of time that a woman must be without her breast and the associated psychological and emotional trauma she will experience. A second operation also involves another hospitalization, more anesthesia, and additional time, pain, and cost for the patient. Some women who do not have this procedure at the time of their mastectomy may not ever have the opportunity for breast reconstruction again.

Again, there are risks and benefits to a delayed procedure:

Benefits	Risks
Time to recover from mastectomy	Time to dwell on cancer
Time to recover from adjunctive therapy	Patient may experience depression from mastectomy status
Time to get acquainted with plastic surgeon	Patient may never "get around" to having reconstruction
Informed decision	Additional cost of two surgeries
Possible improved result	

Who are suitable candidates for delayed reconstruction?

A woman who had a mastectomy at an earlier time, before the option of reconstruction was readily available or known, is a natural candidate for delayed reconstruction. This woman can have her breast reconstructed any time, months or years after her initial surgery. The woman with positive lymph nodes, whose disease has spread and who requires additional therapy to treat her cancer, also is an appropriate candidate for delayed procedure. Another candidate is the woman who wants to evaluate her decision to seek breast reconstruction. The delay between the mastectomy and the reconstruction gives her time to get acquainted with her plastic surgeon and decide on the best approach for her.

What is the correct timing for breast reconstruction if the patient requires chemotherapy or radiation therapy?

Most surgeons recommend that patients with positive lymph nodes or disease that has spread beyond the breast area have chemotherapy, hormonal therapy, or radiation therapy before breast restoration. Reconstruction is usually done 3 to 12 months after the mastectomy or at least 1 month after completion of chemotherapy or radiation therapy.

Some women do not want to wait until the adjunctive therapy is complete and decide to have immediate reconstruction and then radiation and/or chemotherapy.

What timing is suggested for patients with advanced disease?

Once the woman with advanced disease and her surgeon decide to proceed with reconstructive breast surgery, they need to determine the correct timing for this procedure. On the one hand, these women have a less favorable prognosis than if they did not require chemotherapy; thus they often prefer to go ahead with reconstruction without delay. On the other hand, they have greater risk of developing local recurrences, and the systemic chemotherapy can affect their blood count and modify the wound-healing potential. Surgeons usually prefer to delay breast reconstruction until after chemotherapy or radiation therapy. Because some patients with advanced disease have earlier recurrence or relapses after cessation of chemotherapy, some oncologists suggest that reconstructive surgery be delayed 1 to 2 years after chemotherapy. However, the blood count and other variables that can affect wound healing usually return to normal by 1 month. Although each case is individual, the surgeon half of our writing team usually advises patients to complete chemotherapy and wait 2 to 6 months before having reconstruction.

What are the costs of breast reconstruction?

The costs of breast reconstruction depend on the extent of surgical repair needed, the type of reconstructive operation a woman selects, whether this surgery is performed as an immediate or a delayed procedure, and the number of operations required. Simple insertion of an implant costs less than a procedure requiring a flap of additional tissue supplied from the back or abdomen. Creating a nipple-areola further increases the price. These decisions affect the amount of hospitalization necessary for the patient, the length of her operation, and the anesthesia that is required. Costs consist of the plastic surgeon's fees and the hospital charges. In addition, costs may vary depending on the area of the country in which the surgery is performed. The cost of surgery, as with the cost of living, seems to be higher on the East or West coast than in other areas of the country.

Immediate breast reconstruction usually costs less. The patient is already hospitalized for a mastectomy and only receives anesthesia one time. She recovers from the mastectomy and reconstruction simultaneously. A surgeon's fee for immediate reconstruction without a flap and with the tissues remaining after the mastectomy usually begins at $1500 and goes up from there. With the flap procedure it starts at $4000. It is important to note, however, that most plastic surgeons prefer not to do a flap reconstruction as an immediate procedure, because it is a more complex procedure, requiring a longer operating time and having a greater chance of complications.

If the breast reconstruction is delayed, costs are usually greater. Thus, charges for reconstruction with available tissues may start at $2000, reconstruction with the latissimus dorsi (back muscle) flap at

$4500, and reconstruction with the rectus abdominis (abdominal muscle) flap at $6000. A second procedure to restore a woman's nipple-areola, usually costs upward from $1000 and can be done on an outpatient basis. Reconstruction with available tissues, if performed as a delayed procedure, also can be done on an outpatient basis, thus lowering the costs. The usual hospital stay for the latissimus dorsi flap is 3 to 6 days, and for the rectus abdominis flap it is 6 to 10 days.

These costs are approximate and reflect a range seen in the country today. They are offered merely to give women an idea of the range of expenses to be anticipated when considering breast reconstruction.

Will insurance cover the costs of breast reconstruction?

Most major medical carriers are covering the costs of breast reconstruction after a mastectomy. This surgery is not considered cosmetic but is identified as reconstructive, and many states have passed laws to make it a part of the coverage supplied by any company delivering health insurance within the state. Coverage varies, however, from state to state. It is wise to check with your insurance company to be sure that part or all of your surgery will be reimbursed. A letter from your doctors may help clarify your condition to the insurance company. Some insurance companies do not cover rehabilitation of any kind.

Before a woman decides on reconstructive breast surgery, she should carefully read her insurance policy. Some policies stipulate that insurance will pay for either a prosthesis or breast reconstruction and not for both. If a woman receives reimbursement for the cost of her prosthesis, she will not be able to have the cost of reconstruction covered later. It is necessary for her to be aware of these stipulations in order not to jeopardize her eligibility for reimbursement for the costs of reconstruction, which are far greater than the cost for one prosthesis.

In deciding whether she can afford breast reconstruction, a woman needs to assess all aspects of her reconstructive surgery. What type of procedure does she plan to have done? Is it going to be done on an immediate or delayed basis? Is her other breast going to be modified? What is her insurance coverage? Does it cover both a prosthesis and reconstruction or does it cover one or the other? Does it cover modification of the other breast? Many policies will cover prophylactic mastectomies (the removal of breast tissue as a preventive therapy against the possible development of future cancer), but they will not cover what they consider to be aesthetic changes such as augmentation (enlargement), mastopexy (tightening and lifting of the breast), and reduction (reducing the size of the breast).

For women with no insurance coverage and/or limited assets, breast reconstruction is often available through the plastic surgery divisions of university teaching hospitals.

How does breast reconstruction affect survival rates from breast cancer?

Many breast cancer experts believe that knowledge about breast reconstruction will save thousands of women's lives. Some women will come for treatment earlier on discovering a mass in their breast if they are aware of the chance for reconstruction after mastectomy. One expert explained, "This procedure could conceivably have an immense impact upon the entire problem of early detection and treatment of breast cancer."

As breast reconstruction techniques become increasingly sophisticated and widely accepted, more women are seeking information about them. Before deciding for or against breast reconstruction, a woman needs to be apprised of the essential facts concerning this surgery. Her questions should be answered and her doubts should be addressed. This chapter has attempted to provide some of these answers.

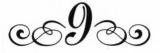

SELECTING AND COMMUNICATING WITH A PLASTIC SURGEON

HAVING MADE A DECISION to seek breast reconstruction, a woman needs to choose her plastic surgeon carefully. Today, one sees ads for plastic surgery in newspapers, the Yellow Pages, and even magazines on the newsstand. These ads, however, are not discriminating and therefore are not the best means for selecting a plastic surgeon to perform breast reconstruction or for choosing any doctor to provide medical care. Many highly trained physicians choose not to advertise at all. Rather than selecting a plastic surgeon based on ads, a prospective patient should consider the following guidelines for making this choice.

TRAINING

The best physician for a woman's needs should be trained in plastic surgery and have met the qualifications of the American Board of Plastic Surgery, which grants board certification in this specialty. To be able to take the board examination, a surgeon must have 3 to 5 years of general surgical training and an additional 2 to 3 years of specialized training in the broad aspects of plastic surgery. Furthermore, he must demonstrate competence by completing an approved residency training program; this means the doctor's peers have approved his moral and ethical qualifications, as well as his knowledge in the field. Approximately 1½ years after residency training is completed, he is eligible to take board examinations and once again subject himself to the scrutiny of peers in order to obtain board certification.

EXPERIENCE

The plastic surgeon a woman chooses should have experience with the different techniques appropriate for breast reconstruction and have a record of successful operations. If he has a teaching appointment at a medical school–affiliated hospital, this association suggests access to the latest surgical techniques, involvement in the education of residents, and awareness of recent developments in the field. It is not enough to be just a well-trained plastic surgeon. A good doctor must know about the specific procedures that apply to the patient's problem, so he can use his particular knowledge to solve it.

HOW DO YOU INVESTIGATE A DOCTOR'S CREDENTIALS?

Getting information about a doctor's training is easy to do and worth the effort. This information is available in the reference room at the local library. It can be found in a book entitled *The Directory of Medical Specialists,* which lists only board-certified specialists. It will list the doctor's year of birth, medical school, the year he was licensed to practice, the year of specialty certification, primary and secondary specialties, and type of practice. Other information on training and hospital and medical affiliations also is included. Doctors in this book are listed geographically, so it is easy to locate the names of doctors in each community. *The American Medical Directory* is another helpful reference, but, unlike the *Directory of Medical Specialists,* it does not indicate if a physician is board certified.

FINDING A PLASTIC SURGEON

How do you find out whose surgical competence is highly regarded? How do you know who is experienced in breast reconstruction? Most people do not know where to go for reliable information. This information, however, can be obtained from numerous sources.

One of the best sources of referral is another physician in the community or another member of the breast management team. The general surgeon is a knowledgeable person to ask; frequently he works with a plastic surgeon as part of a team. He also may have patients who have had breast reconstruction and are willing to discuss this topic and recommend their doctors. Other women who have had breast reconstruction provide an excellent source of information and reliable recommendations about their plastic surgeons; they have firsthand knowledge of this surgery and can personally relate to the surgeon's skill and bedside manner. A woman's gynecologist or family physician also may know the names of plastic surgeons who have performed successful breast reconstructions for his patients.

The American Society of Plastic and Reconstructive Surgeons, 233 North Michigan, Suite 1900, Chicago, Illinois, 60601, (312-856-1818) provides information on breast reconstruction; it also will supply a list of board-certified plastic surgeons performing reconstructive breast surgery in different communities throughout the United States. The American Cancer Society, through its Reach to Recovery Program, is now providing information on breast reconstruction. By contacting this organization through the local chapter of the American Cancer Society, the woman desiring information on breast reconstruction will be placed in contact with a woman who has had her breast reconstructed and will share her experiences. The local medical society is another source of information; it often has lists of specialists in the community and their areas of interest.

FINDING THE RIGHT PLASTIC SURGEON

By locating a qualified plastic surgeon, a woman is not necessarily finding the right surgeon for her. She needs to determine if this physician will meet both her physical and emotional needs. Breast reconstruction is very emotional surgery; a woman's breasts have far greater psychological implications than their anatomy and physiology would suggest. A woman needs a doctor who listens, who treats her as an individual, and who has time to deal with her concerns.

Remember, as with any anticipated surgery, a woman should consider a second opinion before finally selecting a surgeon. Some women, however, hesitate to request another opinion and possibly offend their doctors. They are intimidated by their doctors and are reluctant to question their statements and seek more information. Time spent in finding the right plastic surgeon is well invested, however. Unfortunately, most people do not devote the necessary effort to making this choice. As one woman in our survey so aptly explained, "Most women devote more attention to buying a vacuum cleaner than they do to selecting a doctor."

QUESTIONS TO ASK A PLASTIC SURGEON

Before selecting a plastic surgeon, a woman needs to know that he is receptive to her questions and concerns. To assist a woman in making a satisfactory choice of a plastic surgeon, we have included some questions a woman might ask during her consultation.

- How many breast reconstructions have you done and what type of results have you achieved?
- May I talk with several of your patients who have had this surgery?
- Which reconstruction approach is appropriate for me and why?
- What is involved in this surgery?
- What type of anesthesia will be used: local or general?
- How many different procedures and hospitalizations will be needed? How long will I be in surgery for each operation?
- What type of scars will I have and exactly where will they be placed?
- What are the expected results of surgery?
- How long will it take me to recuperate?
- What are the anticipated costs of surgery?
- What are possible complications from this surgery?

Some plastic surgeons may have photographs of breast reconstructive patients. These might help the patient understand the results that can be achieved for a deformity such as hers.

QUESTIONS TO ASK YOURSELF BEFORE YOU SCHEDULE SURGERY

- Is this the plastic surgeon I want to do my breast reconstruction?
- Does this surgeon seem to understand how I feel and is he sensitive to my needs?
- Has he provided me with enough information so that I can make an informed decision?
- Does he have the necessary skill to perform this surgery?
- Has he explained what he plans to do in terms that I can understand?
- Does his plan for surgery agree with my expectations for what I would like done?

COMMUNICATING WITH A PLASTIC SURGEON

Good communication not only helps the patient find the best plastic surgeon to perform her breast restoration, but also enables her to work with him to achieve the result she desires. Preoperative consultations provide the patient and surgeon with an ideal setting for discussing their thoughts and exploring their expectations for a final result.

A typical consultation with a plastic surgeon about breast reconstruction should begin with an explanation of the woman's concerns and expectations for this operation and a complete review of her medical and surgical history. It is in a woman's best interest to have her plastic surgeon well informed about all aspects of her health and tumor care so that he can consider these factors in discussing reconstructive options with her. It is helpful if he has copies of the general surgeon's operative report and the pathologist's report. He also needs to be aware of the radiation and chemotherapy that she has received, the status of her opposite breast, and her feelings about it.

After this initial discussion, the plastic surgeon will need to physically examine the woman's chest, back, and abdomen to determine the extent of her deformity and what possible reconstructive approaches are appropriate for her physical situation.

Preoperative photographs are a part of an initial examination by a plastic surgeon, and a woman should expect to be photographed during her visit. If she visits more than one doctor, she usually will have pictures taken by each doctor. Sometimes this process is unsettling for the woman, but these pictures are important. The plastic surgeon will use these photographs for evaluating her and planning her operation. They also provide a record of her treatment. He may eventually use them (with the woman's permission) for educational purposes to demonstrate the results of this surgery for other patients, physicians, or professional publications.

Once this examination has been concluded, the woman can again meet with the doctor to review the different options for breast reconstruction. Final determination of the operative plan must often wait until the plastic surgeon has consulted with the other members of the breast management team.

If a woman has a husband, or if there is another important person in her life (many physicians call this person a "significant other"), this individual should accompany the patient for her preoperative visits with the plastic surgeon. Mutual expectations can then be aired and discussed and the influence of the man's feelings on the woman can be observed and evaluated. Even though the man and woman share in the learning process, the final decision about surgery must be made by the woman herself. At no time should a woman feel pressured into this surgery by a relative, friend, husband, or even by the plastic surgeon with whom she is consulting.

If a woman has a consultation with her plastic surgeon before her mastectomy, they should discuss the correct timing of reconstructive surgery, whether immediate or delayed. If she desires an immediate reconstruction, the general surgeon and plastic surgeon need to confer and agree on the suitability of this approach for her. Before an immediate breast reconstruction is done, the details of timing, operative care, and team cooperation must be carefully planned.

The woman who consults with a plastic surgeon after her mastectomy should remember that any reconstructive breast surgery is never an emergency procedure. In the interest of good communication, she may require several visits to her plastic surgeon to answer all of her questions, to clearly explain her expectations for reconstruction, and to work with him to define a specific surgical plan appropriate for her. There are many methods for reconstructing breasts today, and a well-trained plastic surgeon will probably be knowledgeable in a number of different procedures. It is important, however, that the type of reconstruction a woman selects be the simplest and safest procedure which still provides her with the best chance of meeting her expectations.

SURGICAL OPTIONS FOR BREAST RECONSTRUCTION

AS RECENTLY AS 10 YEARS AGO, a woman who had a mastectomy had few options to choose from if she desired to be restored to a normal appearance. At that time breast reconstruction techniques were not perfected; the most a woman could expect was the creation of a breast mound that frequently did not match her remaining breast or meet her aesthetic expectations. Without reconstructive surgery, she faced the prospect of having a lopsided chest or purchasing a breast prosthesis to hide her deformity. A prosthesis, however, was not always the solution to her problem. Sometimes it made a woman feel increasingly self-conscious because she worried that her artificial breast would become dislodged and be obvious to others. Betty Rollins'* humorous yet poignant account of her attempt to find a suitable external prosthesis after her mastectomy reveals the frustration felt by many women in trying to appear whole again.

Today, however, with the development and refinement of techniques to satisfy the requests of women seeking breast restoration, the results of reconstructive surgery have improved dramatically. Women can now choose from a number of reliable procedures that meet their psychological and aesthetic expectations. Breasts can be rebuilt with existing tissue remaining after the mastectomy or with flaps of muscle or muscle and skin (musculocutaneous) obtained from the back or abdomen and then transferred to the chest wall. The choice of reconstructive method depends on the amount and quality of the tissue remaining after the mastectomy, the surgeon's experience with each technique, and the patient's preferences and expectations for her breast restoration.

---

*Author of First You Cry, a personal story about her breast cancer experience.

In deciding which surgical option is appropriate for her, a woman needs to first resolve her feelings about her remaining breast. Does she like the way it looks and want the rebuilt breast to match it? Is she willing to consider an operation on her normal breast, if this is needed to make both breasts appear symmetrical? If her surviving breast is large and she does not want it modified, will she agree to a flap procedure that will provide sufficient tissue to match her large breast but will also result in a back, side, or abdomen scar? Her feelings about her remaining breast will affect the type of procedure chosen and the ultimate success of the reconstruction effort.

This chapter is designed to be a woman's guide to the different techniques available for breast restoration, their indications for use, and their advantages and disadvantages. No one procedure is advocated above any other. A particular approach must be selected with the individual woman's needs and the needs of her deformity in mind.

RECONSTRUCTION WITH AVAILABLE TISSUE

Breast reconstruction with the available tissue remaining after the mastectomy is a technique often used for the woman who has sufficient healthy tissue at the mastectomy site to adequately cover a silicone breast implant (a silicone plastic bag filled with silicone gel and/or saline [saltwater] solution). This method is appropriate for the woman who has had a modified radical mastectomy, with her breast removed but her chest muscles preserved. The skin remaining at the mastectomy site should not be tightly stretched across the chest wall; the surgeon should be able to move the skin over the muscle, which indicates the presence of tissue beneath the skin that can be used to provide a smooth contour for a pleasing breast shape. Reconstruction with this technique is particularly suitable for obtaining a symmetrical appearance for the woman whose remaining breast is of normal size and does not sag.

Surgical Procedure and Postoperative Appearance

Breast restoration using the tissue remaining after the mastectomy is the simplest and most frequently used technique today. This operation normally takes 1 to 2 hours to perform. If the remaining breast is to be altered, this modification can be made during the same operation, and any further adjustments on the reconstructed breast

Breast Reconstruction with Available Tissue

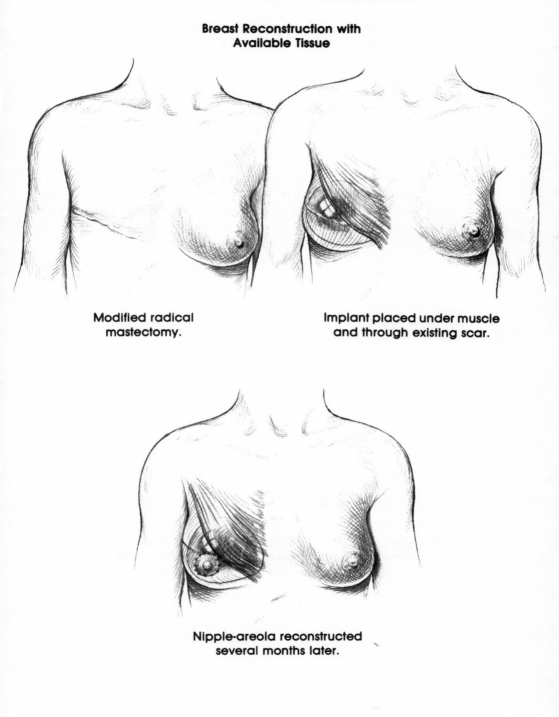

Modified radical
mastectomy.

Implant placed under muscle
and through existing scar.

Nipple-areola reconstructed
several months later.

can be done during a second operation to rebuild the nipple-areola. Anesthesia can be either general (the most common) or local, with adequate sedation. This operation may be done on an outpatient basis or, if done in the hospital, the usual stay is 1 to 2 days.

To perform this operation, the plastic surgeon places a breast implant beneath the patient's skin and muscle to produce a breast shape. To avoid creating new breast scars, the surgeon will frequently reopen a portion of the mastectomy scar and insert the implant through it. He may even remove the entire mastectomy scar and resuture it to produce a better, thinner scar line. When the mastectomy scar is not in the best position, a small incision can be made near the new inframammary crease (where the lower part of the breast joins the chest wall). The implant is then placed through this new incision. Because this inframammary scar falls in a crease, it is barely noticeable.

The technique for immediate breast reconstruction is similar to that just described. After the general surgeon removes the breast and the pathologist examines it, the plastic surgeon begins the breast reconstruction. He elevates the layer of muscular tissue just under the breast, selects a breast implant, and positions it for the best symmetry with the other breast. He then closes the muscle layer and sutures the skin incision. A surgical drain usually is inserted for a few days to remove fluid, especially from the axillary area.

Immediately after reconstruction with available tissue (immediate or delayed) the newly restored breast often appears flattened. This flatness results from the implant being positioned behind tissues that are relatively tight. These tissues will stretch and soften over the next few weeks and months to provide better breast projection and shape.

Postoperative Care

After surgery a surgical drain is often inserted into the reconstructed breast and left in for 1 to 3 days to remove any excess fluid from the operative sites. The postoperative dressing selected should provide the best support for the new breast. A brassiere is chosen if the implant needs to be guided upward; an elastic "tube top" or light dressing is selected if it is to be maintained in place or allowed to move downward. The stitches are removed approximately 1 week after surgery. Their removal usually is not painful because the skin in that area is numb and reasonably insensitive. Because the breast has decreased sensitivity, the patient should not use a heating pad to relieve breast discomfort; she could accidently burn herself. After the stitches are removed, the surgeon may suggest that the patient massage and move her new breast around to keep it as soft and natural as possible. The breast skin may be dry because of contact with the dressings. In this case, a nonallergenic skin moisturizer can be helpful to relieve dryness. In addition, if there are no drainage problems, some surgeons may suggest the use of vitamin E oil or cocoa butter; the patient can lightly massage this oil into her scars to help them soften and fade.

Complications

Reconstruction with available tissue has a low rate of complications. Bleeding and infections are possible but are rarely encountered after this operation. The most troublesome problem is caused by the excessive formation of hard fibrous tissue around the implant—the body's reaction to foreign material. This reaction is called capsular contracture. There is some scar formation around all implants, and most reconstructed breasts feel firmer than the normal breast. Sometimes this fibrous formation becomes thick, the implants become hard, and the breast appears deformed. To reduce breast firmness, some surgeons use implants that are covered with a layer of polyurethane foam. Many surgeons feel that placement of the implant under the muscle helps to avoid this problem because the implant is covered and protected by a thick layer of muscle. They also suggest that the woman massage her breasts on a regular basis to keep them soft and natural in appearance.

If the patient has had radiation therapy or her breast skin is thin or taut, her silicone implant may become exposed through this skin. This complication is managed by removing the implant temporarily and moving additional tissue to cover the implant, or occasionally by resuturing the wound.

Pain and Recuperation

Most women who select reconstruction with available tissue feel that it is not as painful or debilitating as the original mastectomy. The breast area is somewhat numb after the operation, but this lack of sensation is a residual effect from the mastectomy. The reconstruction avoids the armpit area (axilla), so pain in this region and shoulder stiffness are not concerns as they were after the mastectomy.

Women recover quickly from this procedure and are usually out of bed the afternoon of the surgery or the next day and may return to work or normal activity within a week. A tub bath is possible the day after the operation, but the incision should be kept dry and the dressing intact. A shower is possible 2 to 3 days after the operation if all is going well. One to two days after surgery, it is okay for the patient to lift her arms enough to comb her hair. It is possible to drive a car after 1 to 2 weeks, but the patient should be advised not to take any pain medications or sleeping pills that could impair her alertness and reflexes. Before driving, the woman should attempt turning the wheel while the car is still parked in the garage or driveway to see if she is comfortable.

Reconstructive Results

Breast Reconstruction with Available Tissue

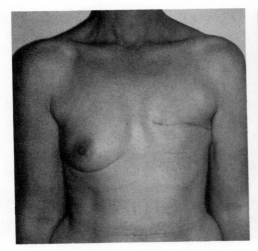 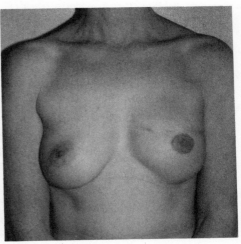

A 42-year-old woman who had a modified radical mastectomy on her left side.

The same woman 1 year after her left breast was reconstructed with an implant placed beneath the available skin and muscle. For symmetry, her right breast was augmented. Her nipple-areola was reconstructed later under local anesthesia.

Breast Reconstruction with
Available Tissue

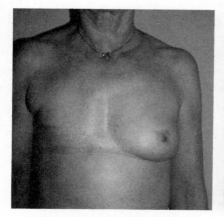

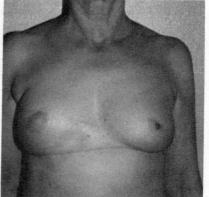

A 58-year-old woman after a modified radical mastectomy on her right breast.

The same woman 2 years after she had breast reconstruction with an implant placed beneath her available chest skin and muscle and no alteration of her remaining breast. Her nipple was created later under local anesthesia.

RECONSTRUCTION WITH AVAILABLE TISSUE COMBINED WITH TISSUE EXPANSION

Some women, despite the existence of tight skin at their mastectomy site, prefer to have a simple reconstruction with available tissue rather than a more complicated flap procedure. For these women the tissue expansion method is a good alternative. With this approach, the taut skin in the area of the mastectomy is stretched and expanded, thus avoiding a more complex flap operation and permitting placement of a permanent breast implant of suitable size and shape. Although this operation is similar to the approach described in the previous section, it differs in the type of implant used and the postoperative management.

Surgical Procedure

Tissue expansion requires two operations. During the first procedure the surgeon inserts an expandable silicone implant through

**Breast Reconstruction with
Available Tissue Combined
with Tissue Expansion**

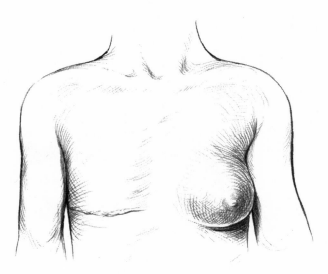

Modified radical mastectomy.

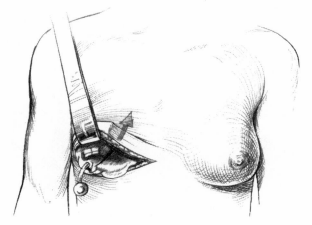

Implant inserted under skin and muscle.

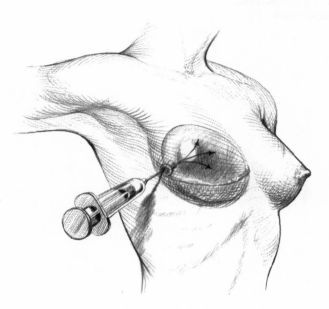

Implant inflated.

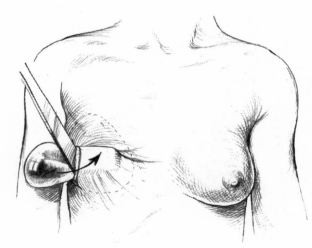

**Expander removed and permanent
implant inserted in stretched pocket.**

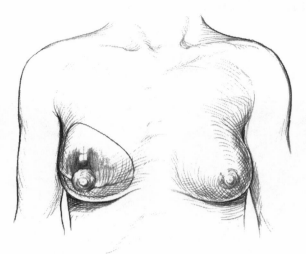

Nipple and areola added.

the mastectomy incision or an inframammary incision (as described on p. 93). He then positions a valve connected to the expander and adjacent to this implant to allow injection of saline for enlargement of the implant. In this early postoperative period the breast skin is still tight and the reconstructed breast appears flattened and smaller than the remaining breast on the opposite side. Once this implant is in place, however, the woman visits the plastic surgeon every few days for several weeks; during these visits the surgeon injects a salt-water solution through the skin and into the valve leading into the implant. This gradual enlargement of the implant produces pressure on the woman's skin, causing it to become tense, stretch, and eventually expand to a larger area. Much the same phenomenon occurs when the abdominal skin stretches during pregnancy. After the breast skin has been distended sufficiently (a little more than the other side), a second operation replaces the expandable implant with a permanent one. After this second operation the reconstructed breast's appearance is more natural.

Recovery from this operation is reasonably quick. The patient usually can return to nonstrenuous activity in 2 to 3 weeks and resume sports in 6 to 8 weeks. Complications are the same as those discussed earlier (p. 94). Again, massaging the breast helps it remain soft.

Reconstructive Results

**Breast Reconstruction with
Available Tissue Combined
with Tissue Expansion**

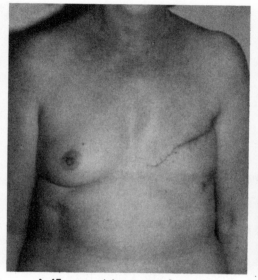

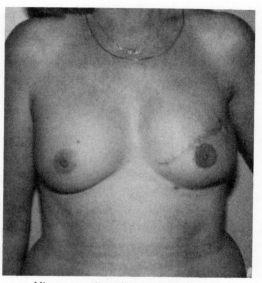

A 45-year-old woman 3 months after she had a modified radical mastectomy on her left side.

Nine months after expansion of this woman's left breast skin and permanent implant placement. To achieve breast symmetry, she also had her right breast augmented. Her nipple was reconstructed later under local anesthesia.

When Available Tissue Reconstruction is Not the Right Choice

Because reconstruction with available tissues is the simplest of breast reconstruction techniques and offers excellent results, you would assume that it would be the best choice for every patient. Some circumstances, however, lead a woman to consider other reconstructive options. For instance, when her remaining breast is large, and she does not want it changed, reconstruction with this method will produce breasts of an unequal size because there will not be enough tissue present to build a large breast. Although she might be immediately satisfied with the newly reconstructed breast, eventually she will feel lopsided and will probably still need to wear a prosthesis to make her breasts appear equal. Consequently, unless the normal large breast is reduced to match the rebuilt breast, reconstruction with the available tissue may not be a permanent solution for this patient because it will not produce symmetrical breasts. The experienced surgeon usually can tell before reconstruction if the other breast will need to be changed or if a flap is needed.

Reconstruction with available tissue also is not appropriate for a woman with a radical mastectomy deformity because it does not satisfactorily restore the missing chest wall muscle (pectoralis major muscle), the hollow under the collarbone (infraclavicular hollow), and the fold produced by the arm and breast in the armpit area (anterior axillary fold). Additional tissue needs to be brought in to reconstruct these areas. If a patient has tight, thin, irradiated, or grafted skin, she also may have limited or unsatisfactory results because the skin remaining at the mastectomy site, even with tissue expansion, is insufficient to cover the implant and to provide her with a natural appearing and feeling breast. A flap technique for reconstruction is a more logical choice for the patient with major skin, muscle, and contour deficiencies.

FLAP RECONSTRUCTION

The use of flaps of muscle or skin and muscle to supplement the tissue remaining after a mastectomy is a major advance in breast reconstruction. With refinement of the latissimus dorsi (triangular back muscle) flap for breast restoration, the results of reconstructive surgery have improved considerably and even women with radical mastectomies now can have all aspects of their deformities filled in and rebuilt. More recent developments that employ the use of lower abdominal wall flaps to fashion breasts offer additional options for the woman seeking to have her breast restored. This method permits reconstruction without implants and with a simultaneous reduction of excess lower abdominal tissue, which is then transferred to the chest area to make the new breast.

RECONSTRUCTION WITH THE LATISSIMUS DORSI FLAP

A latissimus dorsi flap technique is selected when additional tissue is needed to rebuild radical or modified radical mastectomy defects. In this surgery skin and muscle from a woman's back are transferred around to the breast area to replace the skin and chest muscle that

Latissimus Dorsi Flap Reconstruction for Radical Mastectomy

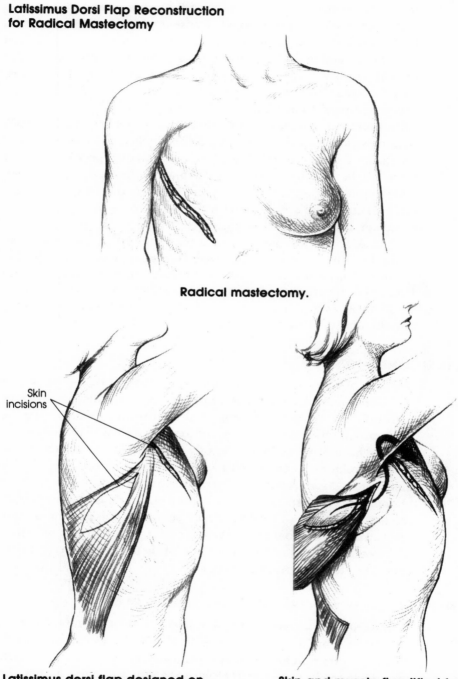

Radical mastectomy.

Skin incisions

Latissimus dorsi flap designed on back.

Skin and muscle flap lifted from back.

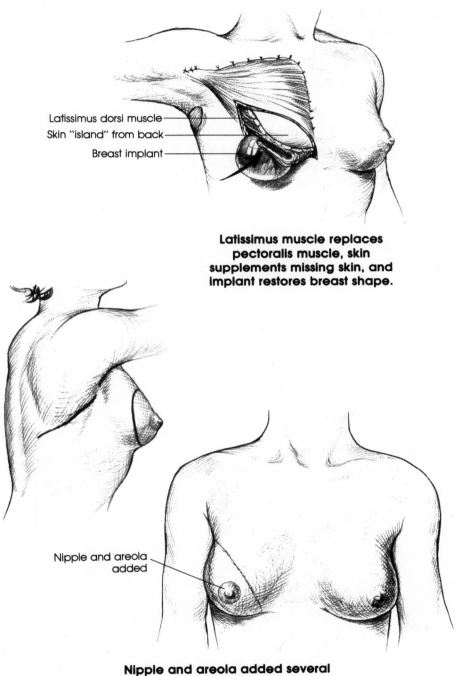

Latissimus dorsi muscle

Skin "island" from back

Breast implant

Latissimus muscle replaces pectoralis muscle, skin supplements missing skin, and implant restores breast shape.

Nipple and areola added

Nipple and areola added several months later.

was removed during a radical mastectomy. This is a safe, reliable flap with a good blood supply. It provides functioning, healthy muscle tissue for filling the hollow areas beneath the collarbone left by removal of the pectoralis major muscle (a standard part of the radical mastectomy procedure) and for recreating the anterior axillary fold. When additional skin is added to the chest wall area, it also permits the formation of a fuller, larger breast than one which could be created by simple implant placement. This muscle and skin (musculocutaneous) flap is also useful for patients who have skin grafts or very tight or irradiated skin.

The latissimus dorsi muscle and skin flap can be used after a modified radical mastectomy to eliminate the need to alter the patient's remaining breast, if it is too large to match with expansion of the existing tissue. Many women would prefer a donor scar on their back or side to a scar on their remaining breast. In addition, the use of flap tissue provides additional cover and a measure of protection for the silicone breast implant. Breasts reconstructed with the latissimus dorsi flap have less chance of developing a fibrous capsule around the implant (capsular contracture), which causes the breasts to feel firm.

Surgical Procedure and Postoperative Appearance

Reconstruction with the latissimus flap is a longer, more complex procedure than the techniques described previously; this operation takes between 2 to 4 hours to perform. Since the operation is longer and more painful than simple implant placement, it is done under general anesthesia and hospitalization is required.

When using the latissimus dorsi flap for breast replacement, the plastic surgeon separates the latissimus muscle from its deep attachments and frees it with its attached skin from the back. This muscle-skin flap is left attached to its nourishing vessel, a main artery in the armpit area. The flap is now ready to be transferred to the chest area. In preparation for this transfer, the mastectomy scar is excised or removed (if it is located in an inconspicuous position), or a new, better-placed incision is made along the lower outer area where the new breast will be reconstructed. Next the flap is rotated to the front of the chest and passed through a tunnel created high in the underarm so that it extends through to the new incision or to the opening left by the removal of the mastectomy scar. The back, or donor, incision is then closed. The flap is adjusted for the most aesthetic appearance and sutured to the front of the chest; muscle is stitched to muscle to replace the missing pectoralis major muscle, and skin is

Latissimus Dorsi Flap Reconstruction for Modified Radical Mastectomy

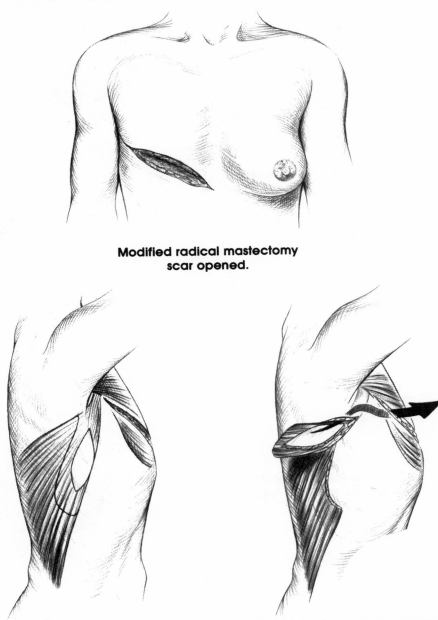

Modified radical mastectomy
scar opened.

Latissimus dorsi flap designed on
side.

Skin and strip of latissimus muscle
elevated on side of chest.

Skin and muscle supplement deficient tissue in lower breast area, and implant restores breast shape.

Nipple and areola reconstructed several months later.

stitched to skin to supplement deficient tissue in this area. When an axillary fold is needed, some of the outer layer of skin and a portion of the latissimus dorsi muscle are brought around and stitched out onto the upper arm. This tissue will span from the arm to the chest, thus simulating a new anterior axillary fold. An opening is left in the outer part of the incision for the insertion of a silicone breast implant to provide a breast shape symmetrical with the opposite remaining breast. The surgeon positions the implant under the muscle to provide a good cover and to permit a more natural reconstruction; he then closes the incision. The nipple-areola is created during a later operation under local anesthesia.

With the latissimus dorsi reconstruction the patient has a donor scar on her back (under her bra line) or on her side (in a diagonal under her upper arm) and additional scars on her breast to allow the flap to be placed into the breast area. The reconstructed breast tends to be somewhat rounder and firmer than the normal breast.

Postoperative Care

After the operation, the plastic surgeon inserts surgical drains into the reconstructed breast and back area for 3 to 4 days to remove excess fluids from the operative site. The other specifics of operative care such as stitches, dressings, and restrictions on activity are similar to the postoperative instructions provided for patients reconstructed with available tissue (p. 94).

Complications

Fluid collection in the back area is a common problem that develops after latissimus dorsi flap surgery. It is advisable for the woman to limit shoulder or arm activity because this tends to increase the fluid. Sometimes fluid accumulates after the drains are removed. It usually disappears after several weeks because it is reabsorbed by the body. When this fluid buildup becomes uncomfortable, the surgeon may need to remove it with a syringe. Blood accumulation (hematoma) in the operative sites of the breast or back is an unusual complication, but if it occurs, it needs to be corrected and the blood removed in the operating room. Infection is also rare, and the surgeon will ordinarily prescribe antibiotics to lessen the chance of infection. Problems with the blood supply to a portion of the latissimus dorsi flap have occurred in about 2% of the operations. These usually have been in women who have had radiation treatments after the mastectomy. When this complication occurs, it may cause a delay in implant placement or the selection of another reconstructive technique.

Pain and Recuperation

This operation is more painful than reconstruction with available tissue. The back and arm areas are sore for 2 to 3 weeks; the pain subsides as the arm regains motion. After the operation, there is normally some pain in the back and underarm area where the flap was taken. This discomfort is similar to that experienced after a mastectomy. Hospitalization is usually for 3 to 6 days after surgery. Recovery time is 3 to 6 weeks to return to work and 2 to 4 months to resume exercise or sports such as aerobics, tennis, and golf. If the woman's anterior axillary fold has been recreated, she needs to avoid strenuous activity with her arm for 6 to 8 weeks while this area heals. This procedure is generally not accompanied by loss of arm and shoulder function even though a muscle is used. The muscle is still functional. It is simply transferred to the front of the body to provide tissue for rebuilding the breast.

Reconstructive Results

**Latissimus Dorsi Flap Reconstruction
for Radical Mastectomy**

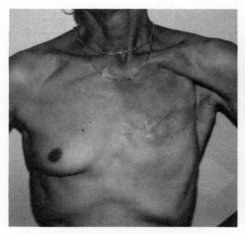 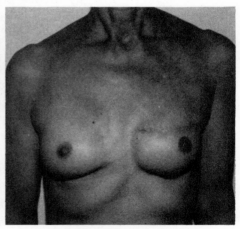

A 53-year-old woman 10 years after she had a radical mastectomy and skin graft on her left side.

The same woman 2½ years after her left breast and axillary fold were restored with a latissimus dorsi flap. This woman's right breast also was augmented for symmetry. Her nipple-areola was reconstructed later.

Latissimus Dorsi Flap Reconstruction
for Modified Radical Mastectomy

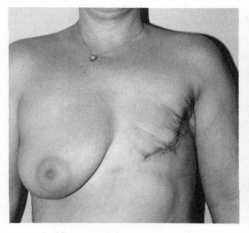 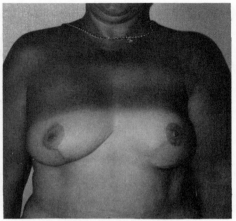

| A 48-year-old woman with a modified radical mastectomy on her left side. | One year later this woman had her left breast reconstructed with a latissimus dorsi flap and breast reduction on her remaining breast to produce symmetrical breasts. Her nipple-areola was reconstructed during a second procedure. |

RECONSTRUCTION WITH THE LOWER ABDOMINAL FLAP

Creation of the breast with a flap of lower abdominal skin, fat, and muscle (rectus abdominis) is a recent development in breast reconstruction. With this approach, the surgeon uses excess abdominal tissue to restore a woman's breast after a radical or modified radical mastectomy. Advantageously, this technique allows the surgeon to rebuild a woman's breast mound with her own tissue, thus avoiding a silicone implant and giving her a slimmer abdomen at the same time.

This *tranverse rectus abdominis muscle* flap also is known as the TRAM flap and is recommended for the woman who requires the extra tissue supplied by a flap reconstruction but does not have a functioning latissimus dorsi muscle or has experienced complications from a silicone breast implant. This is the most extensive breast reconstruction method and the woman who selects this operation should be in good health. Her tissue is moved a long distance (from the lower abdomen to the chest) and its blood supply can be precarious. Delayed healing because of insufficient blood supply is a potential complication. Because cigarette smoking can constrict and narrow blood vessels and precipitate flap failure, the plastic surgeon will insist that the patient avoid cigarettes. Additionally, he might suggest an exercise program for her several weeks before surgery to strengthen her abdominal muscles and improve their blood supply. Sit-ups are particularly helpful exercises in increasing her muscular strength in the abdominal area.

The rectus abdominis flap is not appropriate for every patient. Women who are heavy cigarette smokers, women with scars across their upper abdomen, women over 65 years of age, or those with medical problems such as diabetes mellitus or heart disease should strongly consider less complicated reconstructions.

Surgical Procedure and Postoperative Appearance

Breast reconstruction with the abdominal flap is major surgery and takes approximately twice the time that it takes for reconstruction with the latissimus dorsi flap and four times that required when the breast is rebuilt with available tissues. This operation lasts 3 to 6 hours, is done under general anesthesia, and requires a hospital stay of 6 to 10 days.

Using this reconstructive method the surgeon designs a transverse flap of skin and fat on the abdomen. This flap is surgically freed from the abdomen but left attached to a vertical abdominal wall muscle — the rectus abdominis. Then the donor site is closed. The scar that is left on the abdomen is similar but not quite as low and attractive as the horizontal scar left from an abdominoplasty (tummy tuck), which removes excess abdominal tissue for aesthetic reasons. The flap is then ready for transfer to the chest. In preparation for transfer, the plastic surgeon removes the mastectomy scar (if it is in an inconspicuous position), or he creates a new incision that will allow for a more aesthetic reconstruction. The flap is then elevated and transferred to the chest wall area through a tunnel under the upper abdominal skin and extending through to the new incision in the breast area. The upper part of the flap is sutured into position to give the best contour for the infraclavicular area, and the lower portion of the flap is positioned, folded under, and contoured to form a breast mound. After a radical mastectomy, additional tissue is placed across the axilla to reconstruct this area. The breasts are then checked for symmetry and form, and the flap is carefully stitched in place. If the patient has sufficient excess abdominal fat, there ordinarily is no need for placement of a breast implant. The plastic

Rectus Abdominis Reconstruction for Radical Mastectomy

Patient with rectus abdominis flap designed on lower abdomen.

Abdominal tissue transferred to breast area while still attached to abdominal muscle (rectus abdominis).

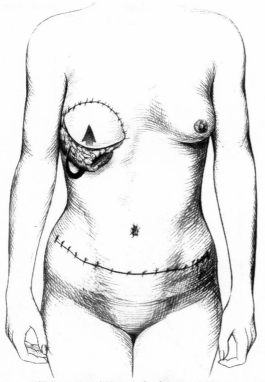

**Abdominal tissue fashioned into
breast shape and lower abdomen
closed as transverse scar.**

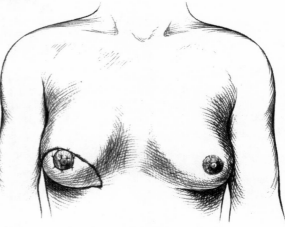

**Nipple-areola added several
months later.**

surgeon restores the nipple-areola in a second procedure under local anesthesia.

After this operation, the new breast usually has a triangular pattern of stitches running along the lower breast crease and up toward the nipple area. A long donor scar extends across the abdomen between the pubic area and umbilicus. The newly reconstructed breast is also flatter than the normal breast. In addition, there is often some fullness on the inner portion of the new breast because of the addition of the rectus abdominis muscle, which supplies nourishment to the flap. This fullness usually subsides over the first 2 to 3 months after the operation.

Postoperative Care

Surgical drains are placed in the breast and abdomen for 3 to 4 days after the operation. This can be a very painful procedure. Because the surgeon removes a wide strip of lower abdominal tissue during surgery, the abdomen is tight and the woman feels a pulling. Her hospital bed is placed in a flexed position to relieve this tension. The other specifics of postoperative care are described in the section on reconstruction with available tissues on p. 94.

Complications

Because this is major surgery, there are more possibilities for complications. About one in ten patients experience healing problems from this procedure, resulting in fat drainage or firmness of the fatty tissue used in this flap. This hard thickened tissue can be frightening to a woman because of its resemblance to her original tumor. It usually softens, however, in 6 to 18 months. Sometimes a portion of the skin edge or fat will have a reduced blood supply, causing drainage from the new breast for a few weeks. If fluid accumulates beneath the abdominal skin, it may need to be aspirated or a small drain can be placed through the incision to draw off this liquid. Other less frequently occurring complications include bleeding (hematoma) and infection. If blood accumulates at the operative or donor site, it will need to be removed in a brief trip to the operating room. Antibiotics are frequently used to avoid the problem of infection.

Pain and Recuperation

The rectus abdominis flap operation is painful, especially in the abdominal area. The patient usually can get out of bed 1 to 2 days after the operation, but it takes another 1 to 2 weeks before she can stand upright.

Recuperation is slower with this operation than with the other procedures earlier discussed. Most women resume normal activity in 6 to 8 weeks, and they can participate in sports in 3 to 6 months.

Few functional problems exist after transfer of the rectus abdominis muscle. Although sit-ups sometimes may be difficult, and women may have to push up when rising from the reclining position, most athletic activities can be continued without difficulty, and many women have returned to tennis, golf, and jogging.

Reconstructive Results

**Rectus Abdominis Reconstruction
for Radical Mastectomy**

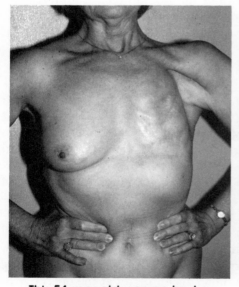
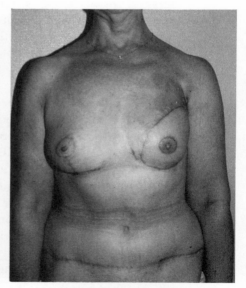

This 54-year-old woman had a radical mastectomy on her left side.

The same woman after breast reconstruction to restore her missing left breast and fill in her axillary hollow. Her nipple-areola was reconstructed during a later procedure.

Rectus Abdominis Reconstruction
for Modified Radical Mastectomy

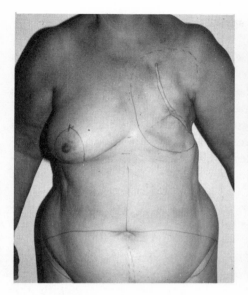

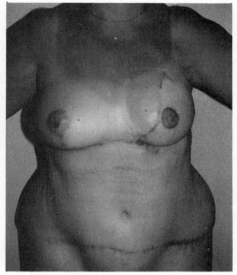

A 52-year-old woman who had a left modified radical mastectomy.

The same woman after a left breast reconstruction with the lower abdominal (rectus abdominis) flap and a right breast reduction. Her nipple was reconstructed during a second procedure.

THE SECOND OPERATION

The goal of breast reconstruction is the creation of attractive, matching breasts. Frequently a surgeon is able to obtain this objective with one or two operations. Any needed reshaping of the breast and reconstruction of the nipple-areola are usually accomplished during this second operation. (A detailed explanation of nipple-areola restoration is provided in Chapter 13.)

Proper timing for the second operation to place the nipple-areola can be determined after the appearance of the first operation is evaluated; the woman's breasts should look as similar as possible. If they are not symmetrical, the surgeon may need to modify the size, shape, and position of the reconstructed breast at the time of creation of the nipple-areola. The need for a second operation does not indicate that the first procedure was a failure. The second operation presents the woman and her doctor with an opportunity to obtain the best possible result.

ADDITIONAL OPERATIONS

Sometimes because of unforeseen complications, such as unpredictable healing or an especially radical defect, additional or secondary operations are necessary. The most common secondary operation involves the replacement of one implant with another to improve the breast contour, size, or position. The new implant is inserted through the incisions that are already present. Conditions of recovery are similar to those described for the initial implant placement (p. 94), but pain and recovery time are frequently less than the initial procedure.

If capsular contracture persists after several operations, the implant can be replaced with the fatty tissue from the lower abdominal area.

After a rectus abdominis flap reconstruction, it is often necessary to shape the breasts further, especially in the lower inner area where the muscle is transferred. Since breasts reconstructed with this method tend to be flat, the contour is sometimes improved by inserting an implant at the time of a secondary procedure.

● ● ●

Today the woman requesting breast reconstruction and the plastic surgeon performing this operation have a number of options to choose from. Reconstruction with available tissue, tissue expansion, and reconstruction with back or lower abdominal flaps are all means of restoring women's breasts. The woman's personal needs and the specifics of her deformity dictate which procedures are more suitable than others. It is very important for this woman to communicate her desires for this surgery to her plastic surgeon so they can examine the different procedures together and decide on the simplest and most reliable operation that can meet these expectations.

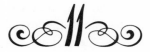

WHAT TO DO ABOUT THE OTHER BREAST

AFTER LOSING ONE BREAST to mastectomy, a woman finds that her remaining breast assumes a special importance to her. It is a reminder of the breast she lost and a symbol of her once unscarred chest. She fears the development of a second tumor in her breast, but she also is protective of this lone survivor, not wanting to alter or touch it unless she has no choice.

When a woman contemplates breast reconstruction, her feelings about her remaining breast must be thoroughly examined and explained to her plastic surgeon; these feelings will affect the type of reconstructive procedure she chooses and ultimately the success of her operation. Both she and her doctor are understandably concerned about the development of a new tumor in the remaining breast, and this possibility should be discussed with the general surgeon. Because the remaining breast will be used as a model for reconstruction of the new breast, it must be carefully evaluated. If its appearance is difficult to match, the plastic surgeon may suggest altering it with an aesthetic surgical procedure. Then the woman has to decide whether she is comfortable with this suggestion.

Most women having a breast restored want to avoid an operation on their remaining breast; in fact, some women absolutely refuse to submit to any surgery or scars on it. Often these women were happy with their breast appearance before the tumor developed, and under ordinary circumstances, they would not have changed their breasts in any way. Therefore, they want a reconstructive approach that will not touch their surviving breast, but will still produce a balanced, aesthetic result. If a woman's remaining breast is of an average size (B- to C-cup brassiere) and the skin at the mastectomy site is not particularly tight, then a reconstruction with available tissue and an implant (p. 91) often will be sufficient to match her breast without performing any surgery on it. Occasionally, the surgeon may have to expand the skin (p. 96) at the mastectomy site to make the breasts appear symmetrical. When the woman's existing breast is large, however, and she still does not want to change it, she usually will need to have her breast rebuilt with a flap of extra tissue from her back or lower abdomen, resulting in additional scars in one of these locations.

Sometimes, the size or shape of the remaining breast cannot be easily duplicated. In this instance, the woman may be willing to consider an operation on it, if it will ultimately produce breasts that resemble each other closely. An operation on her remaining breast is preferable to still feeling lopsided after her reconstruction. In this situation, the plastic surgeon uses one of the procedures applied in aesthetic breast surgery to augment, reduce, or lift her other breast. The final decision for breast size is made by the woman herself, and she needs to clearly explain her expectations to her plastic surgeon before undergoing breast reconstruction.

BREAST AUGMENTATION

If the woman's existing breast is small and flattened, she may want to consider having its shape enlarged to make it fuller and rounder. Then her reconstructed breast can be created to resemble this larger breast. Breast augmentation is a relatively simple procedure. To perform this operation, the surgeon makes an incision, usually under the breast, and inserts a silicone breast implant behind the breast tissue and muscle layer, thereby enlarging the breast shape. It is easier for the plastic surgeon to then copy this larger and fuller breast contour.

Breast augmentation may serve a psychological, as well as aesthetic, purpose by giving a woman an extra boost to her self-confidence during a time when she needs an emotional lift. Fears that a breast augmentation will hide the development of a new tumor are unwarranted. Because this implant is placed behind a woman's breast and muscle layer, it does not cover her breast, which still can be accurately and effectively checked for the development of any lumps or tumors. Mammograms also may be taken, and even a breast biopsy is possible without disturbing the breast implant.

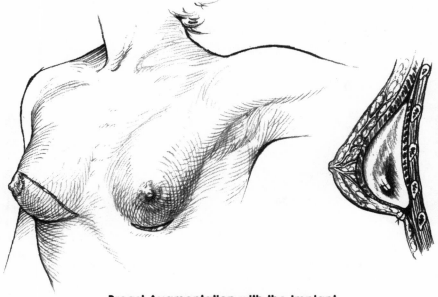

**Breast Augmentation with the Implant
Placed under Muscle**

BREAST REDUCTION

When the woman's remaining breast is large, she may need to have this breast reduced and lifted in order for the rebuilt breast to match it. A reduction also may make the reconstruction easier to perform because less tissue will be needed for the new breast. Many women with large, heavy breasts are only too willing to consider having their normal breast reduced to allow them to feel more comfortable and balanced. In addition, tissue removed during the breast reduction is checked for tumors, and this information helps the surgeon assess this breast's tumor status.

The plastic surgeon does not want to reduce a woman's breast too much; he must know what size to make the breast, because, above all, he does not want to make her feel as if she were losing another breast. Therefore, the future expected size of her reduced breast must be carefully explained and the woman must understand how it will look before the reduction of the remaining breast is done. The decision for final breast size should be made by the woman herself. To avoid overreduction, it may be necessary for the surgeon to per-

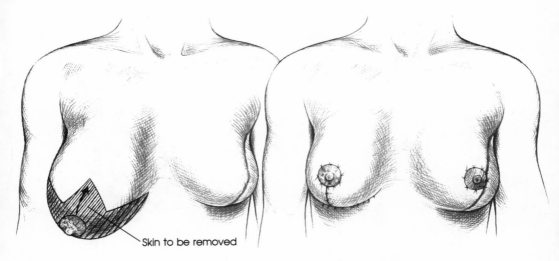

Skin to be removed

**Reduction of the Other Breast to Obtain Symmetry
with the Reconstructed Breast**

form an extra reconstructive operation later to expand the remaining breast tissue. By reducing a woman's existing breast, the plastic surgeon may be able to rebuild her missing breast without a flap procedure; however, a flap should be used if the woman is worried that her breasts will be too small.

The incisions used for breast reduction result in scars that resemble an upside-down T. The surgeon removes the excess breast tissue to reshape the breast to a smaller size, usually leaving the nipple-areola on the remaining breast. Extra skin is excised and the final skin closure leaves a scar around the nipple, down to the crease below the breast, and in a line in the crease. These scars are easily covered when a brassiere is worn. As with all scars, they are often red for the first months after the operation, but they usually fade and lighten after 1 to 2 years.

BREAST LIFT (MASTOPEXY)

If the opposite breast is of reasonable size, but sags because it has too much skin, the surgeon may find that the skin remaining after the mastectomy is insufficient to stretch to match this sagging breast. In this case, the plastic surgeon may suggest a breast lift, or mastopexy, for the remaining breast. Many women are pleased with

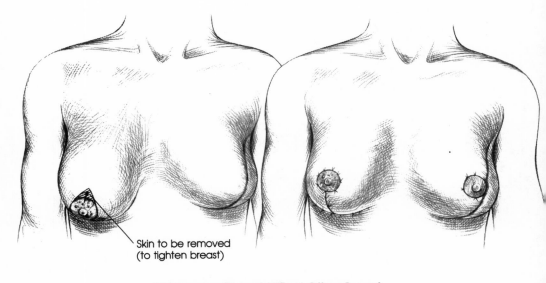

Skin to be removed
(to tighten breast)

**Mastopexy (Breast Lift) of Other Breast
to Obtain Symmetry with
Reconstructed Breast**

the prospect of altering their drooping breasts to give them a more uplifted, youthful appearance.

With a mastopexy, the surgeon moves the nipple-areola upward on the breast to a new position and then removes the skin below the nipple and just above the lower breast crease. The incisions are in a similar position to those used for a breast reduction and are sometimes even shorter.

• • •

Frequently, the reconstructive surgeon can modify the remaining breast and reconstruct the missing breast shape during one operation. The new breast then can be built to match the existing breast. When there is some question about the necessity for changing the remaining breast or when the woman has doubts about this surgery, it should not be modified at the time of the breast reconstruction. In this case, only the missing breast should be restored during the initial operation. Then, later, after the results of surgery are evaluated, a decision can be made about whether the natural breast should be changed or left alone.

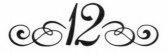

PREVENTIVE MASTECTOMY FOR THE WOMAN AT RISK

MANY WOMEN LIVE IN CONSTANT FEAR of developing breast cancer. Some of these women have witnessed their mothers' or sisters' suffering and even death from this disease; others have themselves fallen victim to a breast cancer. Realizing that they are in a high-risk category for developing a future malignancy, these women are often terrified by this possibility. Understandably, some women seek a way of preventing this disease before it occurs.

A preventive (prophylactic) mastectomy with reconstruction is an operation that is performed with the intent of reducing a woman's risk of developing breast cancer by removing most of her breast tissue and then rebuilding her breast. By its very nature, this preventive surgery is controversial and often raises more questions than it answers. The decision to have an operation to possibly avoid breast cancer also implies a decision to remove a healthy breast that may not develop a malignancy. The crucial question is whether this operation actually prevents cancer. Unfortunately, there are no clear-cut answers. Some cancer surgeons are skeptical about the efficacy of this surgery. They believe that many prophylactic mastectomies are unnecessary. As one renowned surgeon, Dr. Jerome Urban of Sloan-Kettering Memorial Cancer Institute in New York, has stated, "The decision whether to perform a prophylactic mastectomy is difficult for the patient and surgeon because diagnostic methods for cancer are still inadequate and there are no certain methods for preventing cancer."

The woman considering preventive surgery should be in a high-risk category for developing breast cancer with more than one risk factor present. Furthermore, her motivation for this operation should be based on her level of concern over cancer. Is she terrorized by her fears of malignancy and subsequent death or can she be reassured that her breasts can be carefully and adequately monitored without surgery? Most women at high risk are managed by careful evaluation by their physician, breast self-examination, mammograms, and biopsies of any suspicious breast areas (Chapters 3 and 4). An operation usually is not recommended. Finally, the specifics of the operation should be understood; a prophylactic mastectomy is major surgery. Afterward, the reconstructed breasts have less feeling than normal breasts; their appearance is often not as attractive; and complications may develop, requiring additional operations. A decision to have a prophylactic mastectomy should only be reached after extremely careful discussion between a woman and her surgeon. She needs to have her doctor explain her risk status and the full ramifications of this operation, both positive and negative, before she makes a final decision for or against it.

WHAT ARE THE HIGH-RISK FACTORS FOR DEVELOPING BREAST CANCER?

Three main factors are believed to contribute to an increased likelihood for development of breast cancer. Many women fit into at least one of these categories, but that does not mean that they will necessarily develop breast cancer and should have their breasts removed to prevent this future possibility. What they do need is good information about their risk status, particularly those women who fit into any of the three categories of high risk.

HIGH-RISK FACTORS
Family History in a Mother or Sister

The usual risk a woman faces of developing a breast cancer is about 8%. When a close relative such as a mother, sister, or daughter develops the tumor before menopause, the risk increases by a factor of 3 to about 20% to 24%. If a close relative has bilateral cancers (both breasts), the risk is increased by 5 times. When a woman's mother or sister develops bilateral cancer before menopause her risk increases to about 50%.

Previous Personal History of Breast Cancer

The development of one breast cancer increases the woman's chance of developing another new cancer in her other breast. If there were several areas of cancer in the first breast, the risk to the second breast is greater. These risks are further increased if the woman who had one breast cancer also has a family history, especially if her mother or a sister had this disease, particularly if it was premenopausal. In addition, those women who have a favorable small tumor that has not spread to the lymph nodes are more likely to live longer and therefore are at longer risk to develop a second tumor. The risk of this happening is about 1% for each year of life.

Advanced Age

Although recent statistics suggest that more younger women are now affected by breast cancer, the overall incidence rises with an increase in age. Over 80% of breast cancers are clinically detected in patients over 40 years old.

LESS IMPORTANT RISK FACTORS

Women in the following categories have a slightly increased risk of developing breast cancer:
- History of some types of fibrocystic disease
- Birth of first baby after age 30
- Never having borne children (nulliparity)
- Late menopause
- Early menarche (beginning of menstruation)
- Excessive exposure to radiation, particularly before age 20; currently used diagnostic x-ray examinations (even cumulatively) do not reach these levels
- History of breast cancer in maternal or paternal grandmother, father's sister, or mother's sister

WHAT IS INVOLVED IN A PROPHYLACTIC MASTECTOMY AND RECONSTRUCTION?

The objective of a prophylactic mastectomy (also called a "total" mastectomy and subcutaneous mastectomy) is to remove as much glandular breast tissue as possible, while preserving the skin covering of the breast. Because the breast tissue is close to the skin, its removal can sometimes impair the blood supply to the skin and nipple-areola. The surgeon usually will request that the patient refrain from smoking a few days before the operation and for at least 1 week after surgery to prevent any further compromise of this blood supply. Heavy cigarette smoking causes the small vessels in the skin to close down, thus creating further changes in the skin or possible scarring or loss of the nipple-areola.

When the breast is of normal size, the nipple-areola is usually left on the breast and the tissue beneath the nipple is removed. The surgeon then reconstructs the breast by placing an implant under the pectoralis major muscle layer (reconstruction with available tissue, p. 91). This muscle cover will help to ensure that the implant remains soft and does not become exposed through the skin. If the breast is large and pendulous, it will either require a flap reconstruction (Chapter 10) to provide sufficient fill for the remaining breast skin, or the remaining breast skin will need to be modified so that the breast appears smaller and more uplifted. With this modification, the plastic surgeon temporarily removes the nipple and excises the breast tissue and ducts from beneath it. Then he replaces the nipple-areola as a graft in the proper position on the newly reconstructed breast.

After the surgeon removes the breast tissue, he reconstructs the breast by using one of the methods described in Chapter 10. The prophylactic mastectomy and the subsequent reconstruction usually are performed in one operation, even though some surgeons advise delaying the reconstruction for a few days to months.

WHAT IS THE PHYSICAL APPEARANCE AFTER A PROPHYLACTIC MASTECTOMY AND RECONSTRUCTION?

Breasts reconstructed with insertion of a breast implant under the muscle after prophylactic mastectomy are never as soft, sensitive, or mobile as natural breasts. They are also flatter and do not have normal conical projection in the area under the areola, because the tissue in this area has been removed. This flat appearance often improves during the first few weeks after the operation. Despite the limitations of reconstruction performed after a prophylactic mastectomy, women having this procedure usually are satisfied with the results because their main purpose for having this surgery has been accomplished: they have reduced their worry about their high-risk status.

WHERE ARE THE INCISIONS PLACED AND DO THEY SHOW?

A number of incisions are selected for a preventive mastectomy, and the patient should discuss them with her surgeon. Some surgeons feel that they can remove the tissue through an opening in the crease beneath the breast. This incision gives the least obvious scar. Other surgeons have difficulty gaining access to the upper axillary breast tissue through this approach and use an incision lateral to the areola. Sometimes this incision is extended to go over the nipple to elevate it.

The presence of biopsy scars can influence the safety and position of the incisions for the prophylactic mastectomy. When the breasts are large or there is excessive breast skin, the surgeon removes the extra skin either from below the nipple-areola and just above the crease with an inverted T scar or through the middle of the breast with a scar going through the midportion of the breast.

PROS AND CONS OF A PREVENTIVE MASTECTOMY AND RECONSTRUCTION

Although recent advances in technique have made a prophylactic mastectomy and reconstruction more aesthetically predictable, serious complications do still occur. To help her make a more informed, objective decision, the woman needs to question her surgeon about the possible positive and negative aspects of this procedure.

Pros

This operation should:
- Decrease the fear of breast cancer by removing most of the breast tissue.
- Decrease the risk of breast cancer. The effectiveness of this preventive surgery remains a source of controversy. No definitive evidence proves that a prophylactic mastectomy reduces a woman's risk of getting cancer, even though any tumors occurring in the thin layer of breast tissue remaining after this procedure are usually easier to detect while they are quite small.
- Reduce painful symptoms caused by fibrocystic breast disease; however, breast pain alone should not be the primary indication for the operation.

Cons

This operation:
- Is a major surgical procedure, carrying all of the risks of general anesthesia and subject to the complications of bleeding, infection, skin loss, nipple loss, capsular contracture, and implant

loss. Correction of these problems often requires additional surgery.

- Frequently does not produce a reconstructed breast that is as attractive as the original breast. There are permanent scars and a lack of normal breast flow and projection.
- Is associated with decreased sensation in the reconstructed breast, especially the nipple-areola, because of the division of the sensory nerves in the breast.
- Often requires more than one procedure to achieve the best result or manage complications.
- Still leaves a small percentage of breast tissue that can potentially develop a breast cancer, although the risk is decreased.

● ● ●

A woman's decision for a preventive mastectomy and reconstruction requires input from the general surgeon and other members of the breast management team. These specialists can advise her concerning her particular risks of developing breast cancer, as well as the normal, expected results of a prophylactic mastectomy for a woman with her type of breasts. She needs to be examined and counseled by at least two physicians who can evaluate her risk factors and their implications for her future health. *Preventive mastectomy is not an emergency procedure.* Most women at high risk are monitored most effectively by breast self-examination and regular physician examinations and mammograms. A woman should carefully consider all aspects of her situation with the greatest of care before a final decision is made for preventive surgery.

✑13✑

CREATING A NIPPLE-AREOLA

WHEN A WOMAN HAS HER BREAST RECONSTRUCTED, she also must decide whether she wants her nipple and areola (the circular pigmented area surrounding the nipple) reconstructed. Some women only desire to have their breast shape restored so that they feel balanced and symmetrical. A nipple-areola is not necessary for them. To others, however, a nipple-areola is an important component of reconstructive surgery. It provides a finishing touch to their breasts and makes them look and feel more natural.

In interviews and surveys with women who had breast reconstruction, we discovered an interesting correlation between the success of the initial procedure to build the breast and the woman's subsequent desire for a nipple. When the rebuilt breast does not meet her aesthetic desires, she usually does not want her nipple restored because it merely emphasizes a poor result. The attitude of these women is "enough is enough," and they are content to be able to fill out a bra. Women who have satisfactory aesthetic results frequently have the opposite reaction. They want a nipple-areola reconstruction as the final phase of their operation to provide a good match for their breasts. The creation of the nipple-areola seems to complete a rehabilitation program for them. As one woman explained, "It becomes the icing on the cake; it is not absolutely necessary, but it is so beautiful when it's there."

Although reconstruction of the breast and nipple-areola is possible during one operation, the best results are obtained when the ideal breast shape is first obtained. Most plastic surgeons prefer to wait a few months after the first operation, until the newly created breast is stable and symmetrical with the remaining breast. Then the location, size, and projection of the nipple-areola is more accurately defined. At this time the plastic surgeon and the patient can determine the proper position and size for the nipple-areola.

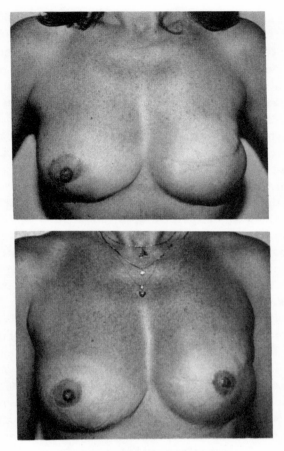

Nipple-Areolar Reconstruction

The actual reconstruction often can be done on an outpatient basis under local anesthesia.

Creation of a nipple and areola requires the use of two different types of tissue transferred from other areas of a woman's body. Tissue for the areola must come from a pigmented area. The skin located in the upper thigh crease usually is selected because the brown coloring of this area often matches the coloring of the remaining areola. A round areola graft is removed from the upper thigh, and the remaining thigh skin is brought together as a thin scar line in this crease; this scar is practically invisible when healed and does not show, even in a bathing suit. After this graft is removed, some stitches are placed in the crease; often these can be dissolvable stitches and will not require removal. The gauze dressing may be taken off the day after the operation.

After this procedure, the groin area often stings and smarts; it will feel tender for about 2 weeks. Sitz baths offer some relief from pain by soothing and cleaning this area. Most women are more comfortable wearing underwear without elastic in the groin and upper leg or panty hose for the first few weeks after the operation. Some women have hairs in this area, but it is possible for the plastic surgeon to eliminate most of the hair growth areas before moving the graft to the chest.

When the remaining areola is pink rather than brown, skin from behind the ear will provide a better color match. After this skin is removed, the woman will have a scar line hidden behind her ear, and stitches will be left in her ear for approximately 1 week. The opposite remaining areola is another place to obtain graft material for a new areola. This site only can be used if it is very large and the other breast is being lifted or reduced. Then the areola can be built from the outer portion of the remaining areola.

Once the graft has been obtained, the actual placement of a new areola onto the breast area can be accomplished. First a very thin circular layer of surface skin is removed to make room for this new areola. The areola skin graft is then positioned on this area.

Reconstruction of the nipple requires tissue that matches the other nipple in color, size, and projection. When the remaining nipple is normal or large in size, it is usually the best place to obtain tissue for a reconstruction. A portion of the lower part or end of the remaining nipple is removed so that the donor area of the normal nipple is not significantly changed or scarred. This donor area usually heals in 1 to 2 weeks without any numbness and little pain. After this nipple has healed, it does not lose its sensitivity or feeling.

When the remaining nipple is not available as a graft for reconstruction, because it is small or because both breasts are being reconstructed, a new nipple can be built from other grafted tissues from the earlobe or from tissues from the upper thigh or labial area. Nipples made from these areas usually do not have as much projection, that is, they don't stick out as much as those grafted from a portion of the other nipple. Even so, these nipples can appear very natural and realistic.

A nipple also can be built from a thick layer of skin that is removed when the areola site is prepared for the areola graft. Instead of being lifted off the breast, this skin is shifted to the center of the areola area and formed into a nipple. A nice size nipple can be created from this breast skin. Sometimes the color of a nipple created from breast skin is not dark enough to match the remaining nipple. In this case, a small graft of skin from the upper thigh will need to be placed over the newly created nipple to provide a better color match. Again, this donor site in the upper thigh area can be closed with a small, almost invisible, scar line.

When a woman chooses to have her nipple reconstructed, she does so for aesthetic reasons, to enhance the appearance of her reconstructed breast. She does not decide to create a nipple for sensation or for milk production potential; these abilities are impossible on a reconstructed breast. The reconstructed nipple-areola also tends to be dry after surgery; the application of vitamin E oil or a moisturizing cream will improve its texture.

A few years ago, it was popular to remove the nipple-areola at the time of the mastectomy and store it as a graft in the groin for use in later reconstruction. This practice has proven inadvisable for two reasons: (1) there is a chance, although small, of moving the tumor to the groin area, and (2) after being moved down to the groin and back up to the chest, the nipple-areola often loses its color and projection. Thus, it often does not produce a very natural looking result. A completely reconstructed nipple will probably produce a more aesthetic result with less risk to the patient.

Although the creation of a nipple-areola is not an essential component of a breast reconstruction, it can add a touch of realism to the result. By creating a nipple-areola as a focal point on a woman's new breast, a surgeon can transform her surgically created mound into a natural and aesthetic breast form.

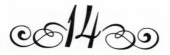

BREAST CANCER AND ITS EFFECT ON RELATIONSHIPS

WHAT WOMEN WANT: MALE SUPPORT

"IT IS ALWAYS HARD ON THE MAN. He stands there, outside, and he sees all of the problems down the road. He is both frightened to death and threatened. But the patient, somewhere along the way, comes to terms with herself because she has no choice."

These words express the feelings of one breast cancer patient as she reflected on the predicaments that this disease creates for men and women. Her statement typifies the type of answer that we received when we surveyed women about this topic. Drawing on the responses of over 100 women who had mastectomies, we have summarized their feelings and thoughts about the problems they encountered in their relationships as a result of developing breast cancer. Issues addressed include the response to diagnosis, recovery from mastectomy, the male reaction to mastectomy, common fears of the mastectomy patient, and male support for breast reconstruction. Although there are no prescribed rules for a man to follow under these circumstances, many of the women we surveyed had suggestions about what had been most helpful for them. This chapter incorporates these suggestions. In addition to information gleaned from our questionnaire, we have also included a short section written by a general surgeon on the topic of the patient-surgeon relationship.

FACING THE DIAGNOSIS

The discovery of breast cancer provokes many fears in a couple and these fears need to be shared. Both are worried about the prognosis of cancer and its effect on their future life together. They worry about possible treatment options and the effects of chemotherapy, radiation treatment, or surgery. Their concerns may not surface immediately, however, since there seems to be a tendency for couples to hide true feelings behind a cheerful, "make the best of it" facade. These true feelings can be damaging to a relationship if they are not brought into the open and examined. All of the women we contacted believed in and stressed the need for open and honest communication.

Women emphasized the ameliorative effects of talking about their problems with someone else. It was crucial to have someone close to share in the burden. Sometimes they just needed someone to listen to them. As one woman wrote, "There is no way that anybody can really understand what you are feeling when you have cancer, unless that person has experienced it himself. What can you say to someone, 'I'm sorry?' Sometimes you just need somebody to talk to in a one-way conversation. Men can help us by just letting us get upset and release some of the tension."

The time between the diagnosis of breast cancer and the selection of treatment is a tense one for both a man and a woman. For a man, the fear of his loved one's death from cancer usually far overshadows her possible breast loss. Understandably, his priority is the woman's health and survival. It is important, however, for him to acknowledge her concerns and be careful not to minimize her attachment to her breasts. Together they need to define their priorities and investigate her therapy options.

The first priority is for the woman to get the best care for her tumor. She often feels confused and depressed by all that is happening to her. By accompanying her to medical consultations, a man can actively demonstrate his concern and help a woman to focus on the issues being discussed. Together they can learn about and critically evaluate the various treatment options. Repeatedly, in both our surveys and in our discussions with men and women, couples stressed the beneficial value of this educational process. As one man related, "By learning about my girlfriend's cancer, we at least were able to understand our choices and make some decisions based on knowledge instead of fear. I actually think it brought us closer together."

THE PATIENT-SURGEON RELATIONSHIP
ROGER S. FOSTER, JR., M.D.

It is normal for a woman diagnosed with breast cancer to react to her disease and to the surgeon responsible for her treatment with mixed emotions. Feelings of desperation, rage, and hopelessness may coexist with feelings of courage, hope, and determination. She may be angry with fate, God, or even herself. Some of her resentment will naturally focus on her surgeon. Frequently, he is the messenger delivering the bad news about her cancer and her prognosis. Furthermore, his treatments inflict pain, create scars, and may deform her body, all good reasons for her to react negatively. In addition to these negative feelings, however, most women also experience positive feelings for their surgeons. Because a woman is dependent on her surgeon, having entrusted her life and body to him, she feels vulnerable and exposed. She needs to reassure herself that his skills are great and that he is a particularly sensitive and caring individual, personally interested in her welfare. Her intense feelings about her cancer and its treatment may lead her to attribute laudatory qualities to her surgeon that are really more reflective of her emotional needs than of the actual character of the surgeon himself.

These conflicting emotions of resentment and admiration are difficult to deal with, particularly for an already stressed woman trying to cope with a life-threatening disease. Her strong feelings are not wrong, but it helps if both the woman, her loved ones, and her surgeon are able to recognize these feelings for what they are. Her anger and hostility should not be personalized by the surgeon and taken as an affront. Similarly she should not feel guilty about experiencing these negative reactions. Perhaps the surgeon has been lacking in tact and diplomacy. Maybe his people skills need some polishing. Even so, a woman and her loved ones need to understand that her anger is not necessarily attributable to the surgeon's personality. Much of her rage is situational, in reaction to circumstances beyond her control. The positive feelings of affection and even adulation that she may develop for her surgeon should also be recognized as situational in nature and should not be misinterpreted by the woman experiencing them or the man who cares about her. The patient's affection or even "love" for her cancer surgeon or plastic surgeon is not the same as the love she may feel for a husband or significant other, where reciprocity of affection is expected. Even though a man may experience moments of jealousy or resentment because of his loved one's seeming transference of affection to her doctor, he should realize that with time and recovery, this affection as well as the anger she feels toward her doctor will diminish and she will view her relationship with him with better perspective.

RECOVERY FROM MASTECTOMY

After a mastectomy, a woman commonly experiences a period of "peak" stress as she attempts to recover from the physical and psychological effects of this operation. Her physical recuperation usually takes 2 to 3 months, but may be prolonged if chemotherapy or radiation therapy is necessary. At this time, she may be weak, tired, irritable, and possibly ill from the treatments. Lifting a vacuum cleaner might be too much strain for her, and she may need someone to assume some of her physical responsibilities until she feels better. Many women said that their arms felt sore and stiff for the first few weeks after surgery, and they appreciated having someone accompany them on trips to the doctor so that they did not have to worry about driving the car and possibly straining themselves. As one woman explained, "My man was there when I needed him most, yet we were thousands of miles apart physically during portions of my treatment. He cared for our children and his phone calls were sufficient to help me through." By doing the heavy cleaning, driving the carpools, or doing the grocery shopping, a man can provide very positive support for a woman during her recovery.

There is a delicate balance between willingly assisting a woman until her strength returns and actually doing everything for her. Most women we surveyed appreciated the physical assistance men provided them during their initial recuperation, but they were quick to resist any attempts to take over. Even though some of the men that we interviewed felt that they could best help their wives by relieving them of all worries and responsibilities, their wives did not agree. Most women were uncomfortable with this treatment. "Don't put us on pedestals. Help us, if we need help, but don't cure one thing and start something else. We do not want to be treated as invalids." Getting back into the mainstream of life seemed to be the focus for most of the women we surveyed. They actively feared being left out of life. They wanted to feel useful and to participate as they always had. They did not want people to "whisper and tiptoe around them."

REACTIONS TO A WOMAN'S CHANGED PHYSICAL APPEARANCE

A man's response to her changed physical appearance worries the woman who has had a mastectomy. Above all, she fears his expressing shock at her missing breast. Many women worry that they will appear less feminine and lovable. Fearing rejection, they desire physical attention, love, and continued reassurance of their desirability. As one woman explained, "No woman is less feminine or intelligent or attractive because she has had a mastectomy, but sometimes it helps to be reminded."

The problem of how to react to a woman's altered appearance is not an easy one. In some cases, the woman cannot adjust to her missing breast and does not want the man to see her. Some of the women we surveyed are "still dressing in the closet so no one sees them." Some have never shown their scars to their husbands or boyfriends, worried that they will be disgusted at what they see. Some even avoid intimate relationships and possible exposure of their scarred chests. In other cases the woman is willing to show her missing breast to her loved one and allow him to help her change bandages, rub ointment on her scar, or reassure her that she still looks okay. Many of the women responding to us suggested that problems could be avoided if the scar were seen as soon as possible after surgery. One woman wrote that many of her worries had been eliminated because she and her boyfriend had viewed the scar together in the hospital in the presence of her doctor. They shared the shock together, recovered from it, and went on to concentrate on other matters.

Although many of the women we contacted felt that men were usually supportive of women cancer patients, not all of the stories we heard were positive. Some relationships ended. Divorces occurred both after the mastectomy and after breast reconstruction. Some men could not adjust to their wife or girlfriend's changed physical appearance or to her status as a cancer victim. They "could not handle the tumor" or stand to "look at her lopsided chest with a breast on one side and a long red scar on the other." Others could not cope with the added responsibility of worrying about a life-threatening illness. Some men found that the woman in their lives had changed. These men now had difficulty relating to her. They tired of "hearing about her cancer" and found her so inwardly directed after this experience that they did not feel that she could talk about anything else.

The missing breast itself, however, did not seem to be the actual cause of divorce after a mastectomy. Sometimes it inhibited a woman sexually and made a man more timid in his sexual approaches, but these inhibitions were often overcome with time. Interestingly, both men and women seemed to agree that divorces or breakups which occurred after a mastectomy were usually the culmination of a long history of problems that had previously existed between a couple. These men were temporarily supportive through surgery and recovery, but then when the fear of death had subsided and life returned to its status quo, the old unhappiness was evident again and often the relationship ended. Marriages or relationships that were strong before the surgery became even stronger afterward.

A WOMAN'S FEARS

Understandably, the mastectomy patient has many questions and fears to cope with. Knowing about her doubts sometimes helps a man to be more sensitive to them. One woman poignantly summarized these worries when she sent us a series of questions that she felt needed to be answered:

- How can I face my husband or male friend?
- Will sex ever be the same?
- Will I be afraid for him to touch me?
- How will I feel about myself?
- Will I be the same person?
- Will I have the same outlook on life?
- Will my sex life be affected?
- Knowing that my husband fell in love with my body as well as me, how will he feel about my body now?
- After I get a prosthesis, will people look at me and wonder which breast was cut off?
- Will people pity me, feel sorry for me?
- If I seek reconstruction, will people think I am vain and self-centered?

SUPPORT FOR BREAST RECONSTRUCTION

When a woman decides that she wants to have her breast reconstructed, she often looks to a man for encouragement for this important decision. Frequently, in our surveys, women explained that despite their strong personal motivation for reconstruction, they still needed a man's emotional support. They wanted to be reassured that reconstruction was okay and that they were not being vain or selfish because they desired more surgery to restore their missing breasts.

Some men will resist the idea of breast reconstruction, hoping to shield their loved ones from additional pain, operative risk, and hospitalization. Judging from our questionnaires we found this initial negative male reaction to be very common. Most of these men felt that the woman had suffered enough and they wanted to get on with life. Most of the women we surveyed understood these male concerns but felt that if a woman's commitment for reconstruction were strong, a man should respect her desires and encourage her. Unlike the mastectomy, breast reconstruction was regarded as positive surgery meant to restore what the mastectomy removed.*

Immediately after breast reconstruction, a woman may not be as pleased with her new breast as she had anticipated. It will not fully resemble the original breast and will bear a scar and feel numb to touch. At this stage of her recovery she is extremely sensitive and vulnerable to criticism. She does not want to hear that her new breast is not as nice as her normal breast; she cannot tolerate negative comments or criticism of her appearance.

CONCLUSIONS

The man's role in dealing with a woman's breast cancer experience is a difficult one. It requires sensitivity and understanding of the great loss that many women feel when treatment of their cancer results in the loss of their breasts. If a woman seeks breast reconstruction, his support helps to enhance this experience and contributes to her rehabilitation. It is not easy being a man in this situation. If he encourages her too much, she might feel that he is unhappy with her appearance and does not love her for herself. If he is negative, she might feel misunderstood and unhappy because he doesn't realize how important this surgery is to her. Finding a middle ground and playing the role of supporting player may be the best position he can take; a man needs to listen to a woman's concerns, communicate with her, and try to understand her desires. His attitude and assistance can have a beneficial effect and can contribute to a woman's return to good feelings about herself, about him, and about the future.

---

*Most plastic surgeons are pleased to see a man accompany a woman for a consultation about breast reconstruction. His presence usually indicates that she is not alone in her decision and has someone to support her.

THE MAN'S ROLE: THREE STORIES

The following three interviews further investigate the man's role in the breast cancer experience. The first two are with men: George Johnson and Bill Jones. These men describe their concerns about cancer and mastectomy, their apprehensions about reconstructive breast surgery, and their suggestions for other men experiencing similar situations. The final interview is with a young, unmarried couple: Scott Meyers and Sheila Andrews. Together, they relive their experiences from the diagnosis of Sheila's cancer, through her mastectomy and chemotherapy, to her present decision to have her breast reconstructed. Discussing the problems that a couple faces when the woman develops breast cancer, they offer insight into the various methods they have used to help them cope with this disease and the trauma associated with it.

GEORGE JOHNSON

Jenny's lump was discovered 1½ years ago during her regular check-up. Her mammogram revealed a possible mass within her breast that had not shown up on her physical examination. She had three other biopsies before, but they had always been benign. When she entered the hospital, the doctor told us that this lump might be cancerous and a decision needed to be made about therapy: whether to go ahead and have a frozen-section biopsy and do a mastectomy right away or come back later for treatment. Her physician also informed her of other treatment options, including breast reconstruction.

When cancer was diagnosed, it was her decision to have the mastectomy immediately. I had mixed feelings about having it done right then, but I wanted her to do what was really best for her. She seemed determined to get it over with, so the surgeon went ahead and removed her breast at that time.

After surgery, the doctor reassured us that the cancer had been caught early, before it had spread, and Jenny would not have any more problems. Knowing that she didn't need chemotherapy was a relief, but we were still anxious because her sister had recently died from cancer. Her death created more concern on both our parts. Now, when Jenny has any kind of problem, no matter how minor, cancer is the first thought that comes to mind, because it is apparently in the family and has been present all along.

After the mastectomy, I tried to be supportive. I must admit that I was distressed by seeing her body with only one breast on one side and a huge scar on the other side. She takes such pride in her appearance that I hated for her to have this done to her. It was painful for me to look at her and know that she was unhappy. The mastectomy had little effect on our relationship. Initially maybe, there was some constraint there, particularly in lovemaking, but it was quickly overcome. There really was no problem.

When a couple confronts this type of trying situation, it's important for them to have a deep love for each other and obviously, after 35 years of marriage, Jenny and I have this feeling. Coping with breast cancer and a mastectomy might be more difficult for a couple who has only been married for a few years because they wouldn't be sure of each other and would be uncertain about what the future would hold for them. I would also think that cancer and mastectomy would be more traumatic for a younger individual because of the sexual implications. If people love each other, however, no matter what their ages or the length of their relationship, they will talk about their problems and try to help each other. If a man leaves a woman over a mastectomy, there wasn't much love there in the first place.

My wife was not happy with her appearance after her mastectomy. She felt that she did not look right in clothes, even though with a prosthesis an observer cannot tell the difference. But, I could tell she felt uncomfortable. When she put on a bathing suit, she would stretch and pull it to make it cover more of her body. Just by looking at her expression I could see how displeased she was because she felt her deformity was noticeable. I tried to reassure her that she looked just as good as she always did, which she did. I felt she looked fine in her clothes, but I don't think she really believed me. Her prosthesis was also uncomfortable and she complained about it. The inconvenience of the prosthesis probably speeded up her decision to have reconstruction. Emotionally, I could tell that she just didn't feel right. She was not satisfied with the way she looked.

I believe that my wife had already made up her mind to have breast reconstruction even before she had her mastectomy. Almost immediately after she came home from the hospital, she started talking about reconstruction and reading about it. We really hadn't discussed this topic before. To get more information, Jenny and I talked with a physician friend of ours who lived in Virginia. At that time, he did not recommend more surgery. He was not really sold on breast reconstruction, and he did not suggest that she have it done. But I could tell before the end of our conversation with him that Jenny really wanted this surgery.

I had mixed feelings about breast reconstruction, but I did not make any suggestions one way or the other. My feelings were somewhat negative because I worried that she wanted this done for my benefit. I also didn't want her to undergo any more surgery with its pain and discomfort. I felt that she had suffered enough. I gradually changed my mind as she helped me to realize that she actually was enthusiastic about this operation and she wanted it for herself and not for me. After I understood her determination to have breast reconstruction, I got on her side 100%.

If a man feels that reconstruction will make his wife or friend feel happier or as if she were more of a woman then he should encourage her, be supportive, and go along with her wishes. That's really all he can do, because she will have to make the decision herself, if this is what she wants done. He needs to talk to her about her needs and really listen to what she has to say. If anything, reconstruction might enhance their relationship. If a husband is totally against reconstruction and discourages his wife from having it done, their relationship might suffer. Once he sees that she is determined to proceed with this operation and that it will make her happy, he should encourage and help her.

In order to learn more about reconstruction, Jenny secured a number of pamphlets, and we read them together to understand the nature of the surgery and the various types of reconstructive procedures. Some of this material was really graphic and showed exactly what the plastic surgeon would be doing and how the new breast would look. It's important for a man and woman to get literature before reconstruction and decide what will be done. They also need to consult with a surgeon together and determine what procedures will be used and what the expected recovery period and restriction on activity will be.

After much research, Jenny got our friend in Virginia to check with a well-known surgeon who could suggest a plastic surgeon for breast reconstruction. We also got a local recommendation for a plastic surgeon. Both doctors recommended the same plastic surgeon, so we felt very comfortable because his name had come up twice. This vote of confidence was particularly reassuring for Jenny. She made the decision to have reconstruction and set up an appointment for us to go interview this plastic surgeon.

Needless to say, we were very impressed with him. He seemed concerned for her and interested in doing what she wanted. His first question to us when we came in for the visit was, 'Well, what do you want to talk about?' This is really how the conversation started. We discussed our interview at great length, later, and I don't think we could have been more pleased with him. He is a gentle person and did not try to push us in any way. After meeting with him, Jenny went ahead and made the necessary arrangements to have the plastic surgery done.

Her breast was reconstructed with a flap of tissue from her back. It was called a latissimus dorsi flap reconstruction. She also had surgery on her other breast. My wife is at high risk for developing another breast cancer. Over the years, she has had breast biopsies for lumps in both of her breasts and these biopsies have been very anxiety provoking for us. Our plastic surgeon knew of Jenny's cancer status and suggested that, when he reconstructed her left breast, he would also remove the mass of tissue inside her right breast and replace it with an implant. He felt that this operation might prevent the recurrence of cancer. Jenny decided to have this preventive surgery to help alleviate some of our preoccupation with cancer.

Jenny also had a nipple-areola created as a second procedure. She wanted her breast to be complete. Knowing my wife, I don't think that she would have been satisfied without going the full way and having a nipple put on. She has been delighted with it and so have I.

After reconstruction, her recovery was rapid, with no complications. Initially, she could not drive for 2 weeks, but the inconvenience to me was minimal. There were times when I had to chauffeur her somewhere, and I assumed responsibility for certain chores around the house that she could not do physically, but none of this was a problem. A man should plan on offering some extra help during this time.

Jenny's physical condition contributed to her speedy recovery as much as anything. She is conscientious about taking care of herself and has always been in very good shape. She was this way before any problems developed and is even more so now that she has had reconstructive surgery. I think she looks great. Until she healed completely, she was limited initially in what she could do with her arms. Now she is fully recovered and participates in aerobic exercises twice a week. She was never confined much. I think she was determined to recover quickly because she knew that I did not originally want her to have this surgery, and she was trying to prove something to me.

Breast reconstruction has totally changed Jenny's attitude about herself and her appearance. It makes me feel good to see how pleased she is with herself. For all practical purposes, she is just like she always was before she started having trouble. She is active now with the American Cancer Society as a Reach to Recovery volunteer. She visits and counsels other women about her experiences. She is grateful because her surgery was so successful, and she wants to reassure women who have had mastectomies or who are considering reconstruction that everything will turn out okay.

Her friends around her age and even younger are all interested in her reconstruction. During our vacation with some other couples, the girls got together and they had show and tell. They wanted to see her breast, even though none of them have had breast cancer. One of our friends who lives in Nebraska and might need to have a mastectomy is very interested in Jenny's experiences. Our friends can hardly believe that she went through what she did, because she looks so good. They are impressed with the results, with her great attitude, and, I daresay, that anyone who does not know that she had the surgery *would* not know. There is no way.

I give my wife credit. She changed my attitude about reconstruction. I really think it's something special now.

There is one final point I didn't touch on that might be interesting for people to know, and it has to do with a person's age and what makes you "too old." When Jenny wanted to have this surgery, nobody discouraged her necessarily, but I think there was some feeling, "Why go through with this at your age?" She was 54 years old, and they felt that if she were younger, say in her twenties or thirties, that this would be fine, but at her age, why bother? But that is not so. She is still just as much of a woman as she was when she was 20, and I hope women considering reconstruction will keep this in mind. If you are over 50, so what! Forget about your age; it really doesn't matter. Do it for yourself if it makes you feel good. My wife did and it has done wonders for her and for us.

BILL JONES

Diane* and I were on a trip when she mentioned that something was going wrong with her breast; her nipple was receding. As soon as we

---

*An interview with Bill's wife Diane is included in Chapter 15.

got back, she called the doctor, who told her to come in immediately for a mammogram. That is how he detected her cancer. He didn't inform her about her disease while she was still in his office. Instead, he waited until she was home and then he called. I answered the phone, but the doctor asked for Diane and he just told her: "Diane, you have cancer. You had better see a surgeon." He was so rude. He just said it over the telephone; at that time I wanted to kill him.

When Diane developed cancer, we regarded it as our cancer; it was a family problem. We were shocked and didn't know what to do or where to go. The haste in which we had to act was traumatic, not only for me, but for her. We needed to find a surgeon and then endure the ordeal of another examination and confirmation that it truly was cancer.

We didn't know that there were any alternatives other than an operation; nobody informed us about other treatments. We went from the gynecologist to the surgeon and that was it: no options, just surgery. Like sheep, we followed.

Diane did not want to have an operation; she did not want to lose her breast. She was really tearful before we went to the hospital for surgery. It was very difficult for me because I don't like to see my wife cry. She did not want to go to the hospital, and we didn't get there until 8 PM, when we were supposed to be there at 4 PM. We put it off as long as possible. She had a mastectomy 1 week after discovering that she had breast cancer.

During the operation, the surgeon first biopsied the lesion to determine if it were malignant. When the results came back positive, he apologized and said he would have to remove her breast. He did a radical mastectomy and removed not only her breast, but the muscles from her chest and the lymph nodes in her armpit area. After the operation, Diane had a difficult time coming back from the anesthesia; we almost lost her. She did not want to live and would not come to. She went to surgery at 6 AM, but she didn't get back to the room until 6 PM.

When Diane finally got back to the hospital room, she wouldn't look at me or speak to me. Then we learned that her cancer had spread and she would require chemotherapy. That was another blow to us. At that time Diane was training to be an elder in the church, and the first thing she said was, "I will not be an elder. I will not go through all of that. I cannot stand it now with this operation and the chemotherapy." The only demand I made of her at this time was that she continue with her efforts to become an elder. I wanted her to have a goal to work toward and not to give up hope. Our minister came to visit and was very supportive; he said, "I'll teach you a minute a day, *but you will be an elder*." His efforts and my insistence represented hope and support from me and from the clergy. I kept telling her, "Don't get mad at God because he did not have anything to do with this." I was trying to fight these feelings myself, and I kept telling her that cancer was just one of those things that we could not do anything about, other than what we were told to do by professionals.

The American Cancer Society had as much to do with getting Diane out of the hospital after her mastectomy as anything else. They sent a volunteer to visit her when she was in the hospital. I still become tearful when I realize that this big organization would take the time and effort to send a volunteer, a woman who had a mastectomy, to visit us just to make us feel better and to demonstrate that people cared about us. They let us know that if we needed help, we could make a phone call and it was available. I think that initial visit got Diane interested in support groups. At first, she wasn't happy because this lady from the American Cancer Society was coming. Diane kept saying, "I don't want to see her. She's just going to tell me that I am going to die in 2 years, and personally I don't want to hear it." Miss Saunders, however, was well trained and she really helped. She was not at all what Diane had expected. By the time she had left, she had raised Diane's spirits so much that my wife was like a different person when I reentered the room. As Diane put it, "Miss Saunders has been through as much as I have. That means a lot to me, knowing that someone else has had similar experiences. She had cancer 3 years ago and just look at her; you would never know it!"

Diane had to undergo a year of chemotherapy, and she resisted it. Every week she would say, "I'm not going to take it anymore." One of the reasons I went with her each time was to make sure that she went. I also had to watch her at home because she needed to take pills, and I worried that she would flush them; I didn't want that to happen. She had a terrible time with chemotherapy; she was nauseous all of the time. She wanted something to help her with the nausea, and we even considered getting some marijuana through the hospital. But, I really didn't want her to take any more drugs, and our oncologist gave her medicine that helped her control the tension in her stomach so that she could continue to eat.

While she was on chemotherapy, we started noting questions to ask the oncologist during our visits. Diane would ask, "Am I supposed to feel that way? Am I supposed to feel dizzy? Is it strange that I wake up in the middle of the night with nightmares?" We questioned everything that was happening to Diane and asked the doctor to provide us with answers. Then Diane developed arthritic pain, and even though she exercised her left arm, it became almost frozen on her. The oncologist had to refer us to a physical therapist to help her with exercises. Some of the oncology medicine was also beneficial in relieving her arthritic pain. All of her problems seemed to manifest themselves at the same time.

Then, came the hair. It was not bad enough to have a sore arm and a breast removed, now her hair fell out. Fortunately, she had wigs that she had used before, and she started wearing them; they helped a great deal. She also got a good prosthesis, which made her feel a little bit more together.

After her operation, Diane did not want anybody to see her. When we were in public, she imagined that everyone was looking at her and that they knew she had a breast removed. She was fearful that I hadn't seen the scar, even though I had looked at it every day. In fact, I insisted on seeing her scar right after her operation. I even helped massage it with vitamin E formula that one of the surgeons had recommended. She would tell me, "You don't even want to look at me." That was difficult for me to handle. I had seen her and I did touch her and look at her; I just tried not to make a big deal of it because I knew how she felt. We finally worked through those feelings to what I thought was a better situation. But apparently, as I would discover later when we discussed breast reconstruction, these worries were still in the back of her mind and she feared that I hadn't accepted her mastectomy.

Our sex life was very bad. Diane was really turned off and the chemotherapy drugs didn't help. The seriousness of the situation relieved me from worrying about sex. Sex was painful for Diane and even though she wanted to participate, she was remorseful and unhappy when we were intimate. I think we came through that experience all right, without any scars or mental damage, because we did not make an issue of it.

I never made an invalid out of Diane; that would have depressed her more. I tried to be supportive, but I still insisted that she do things on her own. I wanted her to return to normal as soon as possible; that was probably the most supportive thing I could do. If a man wants to help a woman in this situation, he needs to return to their life-style before the mastectomy. He should remember what he did before the woman got sick, whether it is a slap on the fanny or whatever and continue those activities. If you socialize, get out there as quickly as you can; get back into the bridge club, back on the golf course, go to church, whatever is your normal style. Let people know. That is what we did. We did not have a closed door in our home.

Our church is our life and it's our social life as well. Consequently, there were many people wanting to know what they could do, how to help. I decided that I would monitor all of this activity. If Diane wanted to talk, then it was fine, and I would tell people. If she didn't want to talk, that was all right also, and I warned them that Diane would explain to them exactly how she felt. That is one way I supported my wife. I told her, "It is okay if you don't want to talk about your cancer all the time. Every conversation cannot be about cancer, and you don't want to tell it over and over again." Anyway, I put the word out so Diane did not feel guilty telling people, "I'm sorry, but I really don't feel like talking about it today." There were no hard feelings and they just talked about something else. A husband has to control that. He can handle phone calls; sometimes a woman is upset and doesn't even want to talk to her husband, let alone somebody else who is saying, "Why you poor thing" or "God bless you." She doesn't need that additional emotional stress, and it helps to remove any unnecessary conversation.

If there are children involved, they should know what is happening. I have seen situations where children can't accept their mother's cancer. They don't even want to talk about it, because the father did not say "Hey, we have a family problem, and we need to discuss it." This sharing is needed before a woman has surgery. The whole story has to be told: "Your Mom is going to come home; she is going in the hospital to have an operation to save her life." Let the kids feel a part of it, and then they will be more supportive. They have a right to be included. Then they can tell people at school and confide in their friends and they don't have to hear it from others. The involvement of the entire family, in-laws, children, husband, sisters, is all important. Everyone needs to be informed and be told about the prognosis. Once they know the facts, the mystique disappears and they can handle the problems better. You can't cope with something that you don't know anything about.

After 3 months of chemotherapy, Diane told me that she wanted to join a self-help group. I was really surprised, and I told her that I didn't think we needed any group. But she said, "Well, I do. I'm depressed." I thought she was doing okay. Evidently, she covered it very well. I had tried to cheer her up. I like to cook so I tried to please her palate. We tried to make life exactly the way it was before, but my efforts weren't really totally successful. Evidently, she needed something more.

The support group we joined had just started; it was only 3 or 4 months old. When we joined, they needed a secretary and Diane volunteered. Knowing she was having chemotherapy, I worried if she could handle this responsibility, but I let her do it. I figured I could help her if she didn't feel right. It wasn't that hard anyway, because I can type, send out postcards, and make phone calls. Her work with the group inspired her and she started thinking about others. That is the benefit of self-help groups. We recover from depression when we begin to think about others. You go there for your own self, but you are aiding others and that in turn brings about help for you. Psychologically, it did wonders for her.

Before Diane developed cancer, we planned a trip to Europe. When her chemotherapy was almost over, we decided (if everything was okay) that we would still go on our vacation. It was a goal we set. If her blood count were normal and she didn't miss her treatments, then we would make the trip. It worked out beautifully. She got through chemotherapy and we were in Europe 2 weeks later. We were scared to death because we didn't know if she would be strong enough. We were in a tour group of 40 people, and they were going to castles and mausoleums and everywhere; I just called time out when I felt it was necessary and we would sit down. Some days we would stay in the hotel and be on our own for the day. She accepted that very well. It was a 15-day trip and it was a part of her rehabilitation, a reward for all of the problems of losing her hair. Her hair was beginning to come back then, and she felt better the second it started to appear. She didn't lose it all, but she lost enough to make her feel very badly.

By the time we returned from our trip, Diane was talking about breast reconstruction. I told her that it was not necessary for me; I was still fearful because of her last operation. I did not want her to go through major surgery. She'd already had two major operations (an earlier hysterectomy) and I did not want her to have to go under anesthesia again. She kept talking about it though, and then one day, she said, "I have made an appointment with a plastic surgeon who is going to reconstruct my breast." When I asked Diane what her general surgeon thought about reconstruction, she told me that he advised her to wait another year, because he was worried that we could cover up a recurrence. I decided to ask Diane's oncologist (a woman) for her opinion. I asked her publicly during our self-help group meeting. "Dr. Worth, why does Diane have to feel that she needs reconstruction? Isn't it dangerous?" The doctor's answer really startled me. She said, "I'll tell you, Bill. Let her have the operation; it's her body." Afterward I started thinking about what Dr. Worth said, and I realized that she gave me a pretty darn good answer. If Diane felt that she needed reconstruction to feel whole, by golly, she should have it. It was not my decision to make. Why should I tell her to feel badly for the rest of her life? It wouldn't make her live any longer anyway. With the help of breast reconstruction, maybe she could live happier. So the die was cast at that meeting.

Next, Diane and I went to see a plastic surgeon. We interviewed him, and he told us what he was going to do. Frankly, we fell in love with him. Plastic surgeons are different from other surgeons; they are building something, not taking it away. It must be harder for other surgeons to have a relationship with their patients. It must be horrible for these doctors to remove a breast, and I guess they protect themselves from getting too close to this hurt. A plastic surgeon puts you back to your normal self again, or as close to that as he can. So it is a happy event, and he wants to build you up and help you emotionally.

I have never seen my wife so excited about the thought of surgery. Just being whole again was all she talked about. Because of her attitude, I became increasingly enthusiastic about her breast reconstruction. Her actual operation went very smoothly. She recovered quickly and in 6 months her scars had started to fade.

Diane needed reconstruction for her final rehabilitation. She has been a happier person since she had her breast restored. The sad times that we had before are gone. She likes to wear a sundress now and work in the garden. She doesn't have to feel awkward anymore or worry that people are staring at her. The first thing she said after her reconstructive surgery was, "Now I can dress and put on my face like I used to, without being upset when I look in the mirror." Before, when I saw myself, I thought, "I look like a little boy." To me she always looked beautiful.

Our sex life has also improved; everything is easier and more relaxed. She is back to normal, and she says that she feels whole again. We have a full life again, and we have gone back to doing everything that we did before. I didn't realize that we had stopped doing things, but apparently she had put restrictions on herself. With breast reconstruction, she is her old self again, filled with enthusiasm. Her zest for life has returned. Reconstruction was the icing on the cake for Diane. It put back what surgery took away and completed her rehabilitation.

Diane was 53 when she decided to have her breast reconstructed. Her age had nothing to do with her decision. Women who are 60 and 70 years old are having it done, and their enthusiasm is great. Some of these women never even considered reconstruction for 15 years and then they say, "You mean I can have my breast reconstructed now, after all this time? I just may do that. I have often thought about it." It's amazing, but their mastectomy deformities still bother them. They are not rehabilitated. Age is not important, and a woman should consider breast reconstruction if it makes her feel better.

Reconstruction has allowed Diane to forget her cancer and focus on other aspects of her life. The cancer experience has produced a great desire in her to help others. Now she is spending 30 to 40 hours a week in volunteer work and I have become involved with it also.

We have formed a self-help group for mastectomy patients; it meets in our home and boyfriends or husbands are invited to come. Many times I'll take the men in the yard and we will talk. One man that I talked to was having trouble because of his wife's anger. He didn't know how to talk to her. Everything he said seemed to make her angry or volatile. We discussed it. It was beneficial for him just to unburden himself. Men need to talk; they also need to express their feelings. I told him that it was all right for his wife to cry; it was all right for her to be angry. She needs time to work through her emotions.

I reminded him that if he and his wife had a normal relationship, she had probably fretted with him before. Yes, as he thought about it, she had been a bit that way all of her life. Once he thought through it, he felt better and it eased the situation for him. Many of the boyfriends who come seem to be well adjusted and just want to support their girlfriends. I think that kind of support is really beautiful.

When our self-help group meets each time we sit in a circle and each person tells why he or she is there: to provide support or to fill a need. Then we get involved in conversation. Someone will say, "I have a problem: I'm gaining too much weight, or, What can I do about nausea?" The conversation gets pretty personal. Soon, if anyone has any inhibitions, they are forgotten. By the time a lady tells you that her breast was cut off, it's pretty easy to talk about your feelings.

It seems to me that in many of these groups, half of the ladies are divorced. Sometimes it's during the divorce process that they develop cancer. I've often wondered if the stress produced from the divorce contributes to the cancer showing up at that crucial time. I do know that cancer strengthens a marriage or breaks it apart. Some men just can't handle cancer and they move on, even if there are children involved. They aren't very supportive.

Cancer produces some terrible strains on individuals and on relationships. Divorces sometimes occur because neither the man nor the woman can handle the word "cancer" and the man runs because he doesn't know what to do about it; he might even think he is going to catch it. That type of ignorance is still out there. Some men also don't like the deformity. To them the exterior, the physical, is so important.

People need to be informed about cancer and the importance of self-help groups. Women with breast cancer need the camaraderie of other people experiencing similar problems. That is how you build bridges. You may come to a meeting and find some other person who lives close to you, and you develop a friendship. You can have lunch together and then you have a buddy to depend on. This person can help you get back into the mainstream and can contribute to your rehabilitation.

Through our experiences, Diane and I have come to appreciate the importance of learning about your options. Today, radical mastectomy is not considered the only treatment for breast cancer, and chemotherapy is often given for 6 months, not a year. There are many positive choices possible for ladies; breast reconstruction is one of them. It is important to remember, however, that even though the choices exist, women are not always aware of them. They need to know the possibility of recurrence and the chances for survival. They should understand the different options for treatment and rehabilitation and know which treatments promise the best chances for survival for each individual patient.

Maybe, when cancer is discovered, a doctor could tell his patients about support groups. Tell them about the American Cancer Society and Reach to Recovery. Let women know what is available. Most women don't realize the type of assistance that the American Cancer Society provides; there are people available who will drive them to chemotherapy and help them get their medication. Women need to know that there are organizations that will stand behind them. This information needs to come from the professionals, and doctors need to acquaint themselves with what is available in the community for their patients. Once a woman is out of the hospital, she is on her own, and she needs some assistance. If doctors want to be helpful, they should encourage their patients to seek help from others. The patient needs to say to the doctor, "Well, Doctor, now that I am through with surgery, what should I do?" Then it is the obligation of the doctor to be able to tell her.

SHEILA ANDREWS AND SCOTT MEYERS

Sheila: It all started when I went to my gynecologist for what I thought was a cyst, nothing big. When he checked me and said, "I want you to see someone else," the alarm went off. He assured me that it was nothing to worry about, but when I wanted to wait a month to make the appointment, he wouldn't let me; he insisted I go the next week. I went to see the surgeon that he recommended; he did a needle biopsy and said he would call me in a few days with the results. When I didn't hear from him, I called his office because I was getting anxious. It was the day of our Thanksgiving dinner at work. I asked the nurse for the results, and she gave the phone to the doctor who asked me to come in to talk to him. I said, "No, that is worse than you telling me right now, over the telephone. Tell me now, and then I will come in later today and we can talk." He told me that the lump was malignant. My head was spinning from the news; I felt as if I were in another world. I was just 30, recently divorced with a teenage daughter, and I had no idea that it would be cancer. There was no breast cancer in my family. I was trying to get myself together, so I went into a private office to cry. I was hysterical and then I thought about Scott.

Scott and I had only been going together for 3 months, and we were very new into our relationship. All of a sudden, I was finding out that I had cancer and not only did I have to cope with that, I had to deal with trying to tell someone who I had only known for a short while. I called him on the phone and told him.

Scott: After I got off the phone from talking with Sheila, I fell apart. When I managed to pull myself together, I picked Sheila up from work and we went for a drive. Cancer was something that I had never dealt with or been exposed to before. I'd never known anyone that had it; it was all new to me. I was scared for her, not knowing what she was going to have to experience. Ours was a new relationship at the time and I didn't know how this was going to affect it and really how I felt about it. I don't know that Sheila knew either. Neither one of us were aware of what was going to happen in the next few months, or even the next year. It was a matter of waiting, talking to doctors, and slowly finding out.

Sheila: When I went to see the doctor, he told me that he was going to put me in the hospital and schedule surgery. Before doing the mastectomy, he would do another biopsy while I was under anesthesia. He had all the consent forms ready for me to sign, because he felt that it was better for me to sign the papers ahead of time so he would not have to wake me to confirm that I had cancer. I signed the papers and went in blindly. I just said, "Yes, yes, yes." I did not know anything.

After I knew that I had to have a mastectomy, Scott and I were just wasted. Saturday night, before I was to go into the hospital, we went through several bottles of champagne, drowning our sorrows. We decided to have a going-away party for my breast. We put on music, got loud and crazy, and poured a bottle of champagne over my breast. Scott kissed it goodbye. It was a wild thing to do, but it made us feel better. Now that I am thinking about reconstruction, I guess we will probably have to christen the new one, too, when I get it. It will be like having a new boat, only I'll be getting a new breast.

That night we just lay in each other's arms and cried half the night. We hardly said anything. We just got everything out, all the tears that might have been held back. We cried and cried and cried.

Scott: It is essential to be open with each other. You just can't keep your feelings hidden. From a man's perspective, you need to express yourself. You can't be afraid to cry. If you can't cry about this, what can you cry about?

Sheila: I was terrified before surgery. I broke out in hives and went white. I had never had an operation in my life. The only time I was in the hospital was when I had a baby, 13 years earlier. I never had a sick day. This was the first time I had been sick, and that really threw me. It had been such a little problem.

I went to the hospital a week later and when I woke up I did not have a breast. It was that fast. They did a modified radical mastectomy, and I didn't even know what a modified radical was. At that time, I didn't know anything. The only thing I knew was what I was told; I put my entire life in the hands of a doctor that I had never met before, and I said, "Just do what you have to do."

Scott: I don't think I thought so much about the mastectomy or her losing a part of her body. I just wanted to see her recover her health. My main concern was her survival.

Sheila: After surgery, the doctor told me that my cancer had spread; I had three positive lymph nodes. I was in stage II of my breast cancer, which I didn't understand. Then he started talking about chemotherapy, and that was another whole trip. Everything you hear about chemotherapy is devastating, and all of a sudden, the focus wasn't on losing my breast, but it was on chemotherapy. The first program he suggested was for 18 months and I thought, "God, how am I going to survive this?" Then the oncology nurse talked to me and gave me brochures on chemotherapy. All of this time when I was in the hospital, Scott took care of my daughter and ran my house. He did all of the cleaning.

Scott: I did all of the housework. There were some habits formed there that are very hard to break.

Sheila: I have a high tolerance for pain, probably abnormally high. The evening of my surgery I took no pain killers and by the time I was released from the hospital, I was reaching over my head. I was determined to block out what had happened to me. "You know," I said, "there is not a damn thing wrong with me. Life will resume as normal." In fact, I ran the vacuum cleaner when I got home, just to prove that nothing was going to stop me. I caught the wrath of God when Scott got home and found that I had vacuumed the bedroom. After that scene, I just gave up vacuuming forevermore.

Scott: That was a good example of her proving to the world that she wasn't sick. I said, "Don't prove it to me, and don't prove it to the world either. You don't need to be vacuuming this house. You don't need to have that attitude." We talked about that for a long time.

I was asking myself many questions during this period, and I was questioning many values. I had to go back and think about the way I regarded Sheila before she developed cancer. I had to determine how I felt and then ask myself why I should feel any different now. I mean, I love this woman, and at the time I decided that I would see her through this experience, just because of my feelings for her; I didn't think they should change because she had this disease. If anything, this experience probably strengthened my feelings for her in helping me give her the support that she needed.

Sheila: He helped me cope with my problems all the way through. The day after surgery, he said, "Okay, let's see what we are dealing with." He just opened my gown and looked down and said, "Uh, huh." I was the one who looked at my scarred chest and passed out. All he did was go, "Uh, huh, okay." He changed my bandages when I got home and rubbed lotion on my scar, even when I couldn't do it. He helped me with my bra, he helped me get dressed, he did everything for me. I was never embarrassed or ashamed in front of him.

Scott: It didn't bother me at all. It was just something she had to go through. I knew she didn't want it; who would? I certainly didn't enjoy it, but we had to live with it. I'm also not a squeamish person. Scars don't really bother me. I wanted to see her scar, not merely from curiosity, but from a real interest in her.

I also knew that she was worried about how I would feel about her body, but it really didn't affect our sex life. We had sex the day after she came home from the hospital. I was worried about hurting her, sure, but it worked out just fine.

Sheila: Even though Scott never made me feel ashamed, I was self-conscious about my body, and I probably still feel some self-consciousness. It's hard, even now, to have a romantic candlelight dinner, put on a beautiful gown, and have one side totally flat. Whether you like it or not, breasts are very, very important in sex and in the way you present yourself. I'm sure they also affect the way he looks at me. He says it doesn't bother him, and it probably bothers me a lot more than it does him. It is tiresome, looking down there and seeing no cleavage.

You have to realize that I had only been with Scott for 3 months when this occurred. There were still many things I didn't know about him. We became very close, immediately, but I still wasn't completely comfortable. Even now, there are times when I am shy about the way I look, and I have a hard time dealing with it. I'll tell him, "Kill the lights; I'm coming to bed." I know that is absurd. You would think that your feelings are somehow attached to your eyesight. But, when you are missing a breast, there is definite comfort in darkness.

Sheila: When I went back to see my surgeon after I had been released from the hospital, I had many questions for him. I wanted to know about the chemotherapy: Who would administer it and would it be done in his office or in the hospital? He referred me to the University

Hospital and to a whole new set of specialists. That scared me. I didn't know these people, and I didn't know what to expect from them. He gave me names of the doctors at the hospital and handed me my pathology report in a sealed envelope.

I went home and immediately ripped open the report and read through it. I came to the part that said, "Prognosis: poor" and I went bing! I had no business reading that report. I didn't know what I was reading and I did not know how to interpret it. It scared the hell out of me.

Scott: We both read through the pathology report, but I didn't understand most of it, only words here and there. At the bottom, it read: "Prognosis: condition poor." That, everyone can read; it was black and white and simple language. It was also very difficult to take. We had both just been through her surgery and were trying to remain positive. Then to have something like that come along is demoralizing. It is like having someone tell you that all of your effort is not worth shit; it doesn't matter what you do, because this is the way it is.

Sheila: Six weeks after my surgery, I went to the hospital to see the doctors about chemotherapy. They told me that the type of cancer I had was poorly differentiated and had a high recurrence rate. That was another blow. I went into a rage. I cursed them and screamed, "Bullshit. You are not telling me that I am dying. I am only 30 years old. I have a daughter and my own house. For the first time in my life, after a terrible marriage, I have a man that I really love; I have everything to live for: a new job, a new relationship, a child, everything." I really fought it, and I've continued to fight it. I have bad moods, but I am not going to let it get me.

Scott: I think the chemotherapy was even more of an adjustment for Sheila than the surgery itself. Chemotherapy required a great deal of patience and understanding from me and from everyone around Sheila, especially her daughter. The drugs affected her poorly. She was moody and short-fused. She had a temper and she cried all of the time. She stayed in bed a lot. I could deal with that and her daughter handled it well. Her daughter showed real understanding and patience for her mother and what she was enduring; I think she knew that Sheila was not always going to act that way and there would be an end to it. We were all relieved when the chemotherapy was over. It really pushed everyone to the maximum. I had to keep telling myself that the drugs were making her react the way she was.

She said many dumb things during that time. I think her logic and reasoning were not as clear as they normally were, and she was very emotional.

Sheila: You go through so many emotions with cancer, and chemotherapy does trigger those emotions. You are high at one moment and then lower than a snake the next. My moods were up and down. I don't think I was really rational for many of the things that I did or said. I wasn't altogether there and I wasn't in control all of the time. Despite my actions and the way life was treating me, Scott moved in with me during my chemotherapy. I really knew he loved me if he could move in at that time.

Chemotherapy was terrible for me. I had very long, luscious blonde hair and after the first chemotherapy treatment, it started coming out in handfuls. During the second week, I had big clumps of hair falling out of my head. I made an appointment to see wigs and they matched me with several long, blonde wigs. Soon, I was practically bald. I looked like Bozo the Clown; I had a strip of hair running along the edges of my scalp. I not only lost the hair on my head, but I also lost the rest of my body hair, every bit, from head to toe. I still had a few eyelashes, but my eyebrows were almost nonexistent. I had to wear a lot of makeup to look normal. I also gained 18 pounds on chemotherapy, which I am having a hard time losing. So, besides being bald, not getting into my clothes, and losing a breast, I kept saying, "What is next?" It is a tremendous amount to deal with.

Scott: Hair loss was traumatic for Sheila. She seemed to have an enormous amount to cope with, and it was sometimes hard for me to help her.

Sheila: With a breast, you can camouflage your loss, but with hair loss, what can you do? I mean, I couldn't wear wigs to bed. Talk about romance. He had to look at this woman who had one breast and was bald as a billiard ball. "Oh my God, I looked like I just stepped out of a circus." We can laugh now, but at the time there were many tears. Finally, all this hair was falling out and he made the ultimate decision. He said, "Sheila, you are clogging all of the drains. I have to cut off every bit of your hair, because it is falling out, and it is getting all over your clothes. Let's just get it over with once and for all." I said, "Okay," and he got the scissors and just snipped off the rest; that was probably the best thing he ever did. He just got rid of it, and I stopped worrying about it falling out.

Scott: There were times when I needed someone to confide in. I have one or two close friends that I can talk to, but they didn't really understand what was happening.

Sheila: We often talked about our relationship. In fact, there were times when we weren't sure that it would last. It had nothing to do with my cancer, it was just his own feelings. He has other commitments; he goes to school, he works, and he loves to travel. It's hard to commit yourself to a woman who has cancer, who is going through chemotherapy, and who has a 13-year-old daughter and a house. That's a lot to ask of anyone. He had to be absolutely sure how he felt about me before he made any kind of commitment to me.

Scott: I needed to work through my own feelings and think about my life. I thought about how I felt about Sheila before surgery and before she had cancer. I had to decide what I was feeling now. I had to confront myself: "Am I staying with this woman because I pity her or because I love her?" There were times when I really couldn't answer that question. Finally, I decided that if I left I would never know and if I stayed, I would have to be very careful about why I stayed. I decided that I wanted to stay. I love her and I wanted to give her 100% of my support and love and see her through this experience. If there were anything that I could do to help her, I would do it. That meant taking care of her, her surroundings, and her daughter. It meant providing moral support and letting her know that she was going to get through this okay. I was determined to keep as optimistic an attitude as I could and to show some strength for her.

Sheila: He was always planning for the future. That was important for me because when all of this first happened, I didn't take any interest in the house or even in balancing the checkbook. I owned my own house, and we talked about painting it. But I would say things like, "Why should I paint this damn place if I am going to die? Why should I buy anything?" I didn't want to buy anything: clothes, furniture, paint, anything. Why should I, if I weren't going to be able to enjoy it in 6 months? Toward the end of my chemotherapy, many of these feelings disappeared; we repainted the house, and I started buying clothes again.

Scott: She started living a normal life again. She joined a support group through the American Cancer Society and she started taking dancing lessons. By remembering that there were other things that she needed to do with her life, she began to get out again and not let this hold her back.

Sheila: You can allow yourself to get depressed and let everyone feel sorry for you. It's easy to have a sad face and then people will say, "Oh, I'm so sorry." I didn't want that crap. I just wanted to be happy and to laugh. Scott and I had funny experiences and we tried to keep our sense of humor. Our laughter has helped me survive this experience. When I go to my support group, I tell people about the funny things that happen. Like the time I forgot to put the toilet seat down and my wig fell in. I had to shake it out, wash it, and hang it out in the sun to dry. Then I realized that I couldn't go anywhere, because I was bald, my other wig was being fixed, and I only had this one. You must laugh at things like that.

Scott: I wanted to take her to a loud dance studio in town, with her dressed like the lady in Star Trek. She wouldn't have it.

Sheila: He wanted to dress me in silver tights and makeup. He wanted me to be a Trekkie. He told me it would be the chance of a lifetime.

Actually, we did have fun with it. We went to a Kenny Loggins concert in June and I was still pretty bald at the time. I had ⅛ inch of hair all over my head so I decided to dress in style. I bought myself a bright lavender headband and put on a black jumpsuit with high heels and makeup. I wore lavender and black jewelry, earrings that were as big as my head, and beads. I didn't wear my wig. We went to the concert and people did double and triple takes. I'm sure they were talking about that bald woman. "A good-looking man like that with a bald woman, yuck!" It was really interesting. The women made derogatory comments about my head, but the men seemed to be complimentary. It was very, very strange. If they had only known why I looked the way I did.

Getting involved with support groups has also helped me to adjust. Women need to know that there are self-help groups available and that we are not alone. The American Cancer Society has a number of these groups going. Reach to Recovery is one and I am now a volunteer. I'm also in another support group that meets once a month and we swap stories about our experiences. It's one of those meetings where you can cry, especially with the women who have just come out of it. We cry, we hold each other, we laugh. You can face a lot of things together.

One of the women in our group just had a recurrence. She had her surgery the same time I did, and she was just getting ready for her yearly checkup when they found an inoperable mass in her chest. She only has 6 months to live. You have to learn that when you are working closely with people, not everyone is going to make it and that's hard to take. I had to come to grips with that reality this month with her.

We share everything in these meetings. We talk about sex and looks and feelings. Many of these women are single and are dating. They ask, "How do you tell a man that you've had this surgery? Maybe you've only gone out with him two or three times, and it gets to a point where you might end up in bed. What do you do then?" That's a problem that you need to broach and you need to know what to do. Even with Scott it was difficult for me because I was still self-conscious.

I learned about breast reconstruction in my support group. One of the women had it done and she told me about her plastic surgeon. I had no idea that there were any alternatives. My surgeon never said anything about reconstruction. After I heard about it though, halfway through my chemotherapy, I started asking doctors at the hospital about breast reconstruction, and they said, "Go for it." They were very supportive. But they also told me that I would have to wait until the chemotherapy was over. Then they said, "Do it. You're young and you want your breast back. It would be a great thing for your mental attitude."

Scott: I really didn't like the idea of her doing it. I'm not comfortable with it. I don't want her going into an operating room again. We have talked about it quite a bit, and I am concerned because I feel that she is doing this entirely for me, and there is no need.

Sheila: Probably he is right to a certain extent. I am doing this partly for him, but it is also for me. I think that if I have breast reconstruction, I'll feel better about myself and the way that I look. After a mastectomy, every time that you look at yourself in the mirror, it's a reminder of cancer. Personally, I don't feel I have cancer anymore; I really don't. It's something I had to deal with at the time, but now it is time to go ahead and get my breast reconstructed and stop worrying about it. I don't want to look down any more and see that there is a breast missing. I miss wearing regular bathing suits and nice lingerie. Actually, the more I think about it, the more I realize that I am doing it for myself. It is to help me forget this disease.

I like to sleep on my stomach, but with a missing breast this position becomes awkward and off balance. I am also uncomfortable with my prosthesis. I'm an accountant and just moving my arm to the calculator makes the prosthesis rub; it bothers me. The first thing I do when I get home from work is kick off my shoes and throw out my prosthesis.

In my mind, I made a commitment to investigate breast reconstruction the minute I heard that it was a possibility. I decided that I wanted it if I could have it.

I was really scared when I went to see the plastic surgeon. The first time he saw me, he told me to take off my clothes so he could take some photos. He got out his camera and took about 20 pictures of every angle of my breast. He was also taking pictures of my stomach and my hips. Meanwhile, I'm thinking, "Oh my God. Blackmail!" I felt like I was posing for *Playboy*. But he needed those pictures to decide what to do, and he said that with the weight I had gained during chemotherapy and after having had a child, he felt an abdominal flap was the best operation for me. You see, I don't have an 18-year-old stomach anymore, and yet my remaining breast has a nice size and shape. If I had this flap surgery he wouldn't have to touch my opposite breast. He felt he could get the best match for my breast with an abdominal flap reconstruction; and I would be more pleased with it, knowing that I could get rid of my stomach and also get a breast to match my remaining breast.

I had to think a long time about having this operation. Not only am I going in for more surgery, but I am having a major operation; this is the most complicated form of reconstruction. It is a big deal to decide. When you have cancer, you don't have a choice. You go into the hospital, and you get surgery. I'm going into a major operation that is by choice and that is hard. I am saying, "Okay, Doc, I'm going to let you rearrange my entire body and I'm putting it in your hands." If I didn't trust my plastic surgeon, I wouldn't be able to say that. It shows you how much faith I have in him. I am saying, "Do your best. I totally trust you with my life."

Scott: She isn't making this decision based on ignorance, however. Since her mastectomy, we've taken time to learn about reconstruction.

Sheila: Several weeks ago we invited a girl over to our house. She had this same operation by another surgeon, and we wanted to see somebody else's work. She came over 8 weeks after her surgery and she showed Scott and me her breast. She just stripped down and said, "Okay, this is what I look like." It was nice seeing another breast. When you go into this, you have to understand that your body is

never going to look exactly the same as it did before. There are going to be some concessions. There are going to be some scars; I will
have a scar across my stomach. My main concern is my appearance
in clothes; now I will be able to wear a bra and will not have to wear
a prosthesis. I will be able to fill something out again."

Scott: I'm still having problems with her having more surgery. It's
another operation and it worries me. But if it's going to help her
psychologically and improve her self-image, then I want her to have
it. It has to be important to her.

Sheila: I am looking forward to breast reconstruction. I am not interested in having a nipple-areola put on right now; it's not a priority
for me. I've heard that it is an uncomfortable procedure, and I told
my plastic surgeon that I will wait until he perfects things a little
better. I can always go in later and have it put on. I'm not in a
hurry. No one would really see the nipple, except Scott. If I feel
deprived, I can probably just cut out brown construction paper and
stick it on.

I want to be able to wear a normal bathing suit this summer. In
fact, the night before my surgery I'm meeting my plastic surgeon at
the hospital with my bathing suit. It has a French cut to the legs and
instead of a straight line cut across my abdomen, he is going to give
me a "happy face" scar so that I can still wear this suit. I'm going to
try on my suit for him so he can plan my scars to fall in the right
area. Women don't understand that the scar doesn't have to extend
straight from hip to hip; it can be curved up. It's nice to know that
even these details can be individualized.

Women need to know about breast reconstruction and about the
different options for cancer treatment. They need this information
before it happens to them. Every woman should be informed about
breast cancer. She should know about mastectomies and reconstruction before she has to worry about them. I went into this experience so ignorant. I just said, "Do what you want." I didn't know anything. I didn't know that there were alternatives; I didn't know that
there was breast reconstruction. I think if women knew about reconstruction and knew the results, they might not be so hesitant to go in
if they felt a lump. I really think that detection is the key, and
knowledge about alternatives and treatment will encourage women
to report problems as soon as they discover them.

Scott: I agree with Sheila 100%. I think women should be educated.
They should know their options, and they should get involved in

them. Once you've experienced what we have experienced, you learn to be happy and to make the most of life. You learn that one of the most effective ways of coping with a situation like this is by remaining positive.

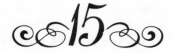

Eight Women Tell Their Stories

IN THE PROCESS OF WRITING this book, we were assisted by many women who sensitively and generously communicated their thoughts and feelings to us. Their help has been invaluable and what they have shared has both touched and motivated us to try to give you some insights into their situations. Following are eight different stories of women who had mastectomies for breast cancer and sought breast reconstruction. We have altered the names and personal details for each of these women to protect their privacy.

We have purposely selected women who had different reconstructive procedures performed, to give you some idea of the reconstructive possibilities available with their potential benefits and problems. These women range in age from 27 to 63 and represent every social and cultural background. In addition, the questions we asked varied from woman to woman in order to provide wider coverage of topics. Thus, one story focuses on the issues of vanity and self-image for the woman seeking breast restoration; whereas another explains the problems that the woman with a mastectomy faces in dating. Certain subjects, however, are dealt with in each dialogue, including reasons for deciding on breast reconstruction, timing of reconstructive surgery, pain and recuperation after reconstruction, physical and psychological results of reconstructive surgery, and benefits and limitations of reconstructive surgery. An attempt has been made to present an honest, well-rounded discussion of this option so that women contemplating reconstructive surgery will have a realistic understanding of what this surgery might offer them.

Because the female half of this writing team did most of the first-hand interviewing, in order to provide an avenue for free discussion between women, these stories and the questions and observations are presented in the first person.

ELLEN: A QUESTION OF VANITY

"It seems that we are bombarded by advertisements that say that we have to be voluptuous and beautiful, and then one day we sit across from a man who says, 'Well, in order to save your life, we are going to remove your breast.' Then you reply, 'But I just turned on the TV and it says that to be desirable I have to have two breasts and be beautiful and you're telling me it doesn't matter.' You are trying to decide what to do, and he is telling you that it is vanity (at least I thought it was vanity at one point) to want to keep your breasts. I thought it would be vain of me to even consider not having a mastectomy, especially when my surgeon told me that I had to have one, and it would be vain to even think about reconstruction."

These poignant comments were made to me by Ellen as we discussed her experiences with mastectomy and reconstruction. Ellen is a strikingly attractive 39-year-old woman. When I first saw her she was waiting by the hospital elevator on her way to our interview. I casually admired her figure, the way one woman appraises another, and was impressed with her style and demeanor. When I actually met her, I was surprised to learn that she was one of the breast reconstruction patients whom I was to interview. Ellen is intelligent and introspective. She has carefully analyzed her feelings about her mastectomy and her reconstructive breast surgery. Married with two children, Ellen had a radical mastectomy on her left breast 5 years ago; this surgery left her with "a diagonal scar from her shoulder across her chest and a concavity just below the clavicle." "I really looked like a scrub board. Not only was I missing a breast, but you could count my ribs; they stuck out so prominently. I definitely needed filling in if I were ever to appear normal again."

Two years ago Ellen decided to have breast reconstruction. One of the biggest obstacles she faced in reaching this decision concerned the question of vanity. Following are more excerpts from my conversation with Ellen.

Why did you decide you wanted to have your breast reconstructed?

My mental attitude after the mastectomy was that I probably wouldn't have it done. I was trying to feel good about myself again, which took a little while. Then I thought that I didn't need it. I was functioning very nicely without it, thank you. At the time I thought I still had to be strong and deal with this thing and still be the same wife and the same mother and the same everything, and it was ridiculous. Nobody expected that, except me. Certainly not my husband, certainly not my sons. I felt I had to do this.

Then, I started to pick up an article here and an article there on breast reconstruction and every time I turned on the TV there was Phil Donahue or someone else talking about the same subject. And I would think about it, and I would say, "Gosh, I don't know. Maybe people will think I'm vain, or they will think: Why did she do that? She was perfectly fine the way she was." I guess I cared that much for what other people thought, and I thought I had to be superwoman and did not need this.

Even 3 years after the mastectomy, when I consulted with a plastic surgeon about my reconstruction, I wasn't dying to have this operation. I rationalized my decision for more surgery because of the physical problems I was having. I had developed backaches. I wear a C cup so my prosthesis had some weight to it; it bothered my back, and it was so hot and such an annoyance in the summer. I was very rational about this whole subject. "Certainly, I told myself, reconstruction is something you want, just because of the prosthesis and to make your back feel better." So I decided to go ahead for those reasons.

Later, however, after I started to cope with what I had done and looked at myself in the mirror, I realized that, to be totally honest, I wanted to look good again, and I wanted to wear a bathing suit again, and I wanted to feel sexy again. These were all things that in my heart I expected and cared about. These were things that I wanted for myself, but I didn't know it then. I did not know it until afterward, when I started to dress normally and could get up in the morning and forget that I had had a mastectomy. I looked wonderful. Then I realized how important it was. It was the best thing that could have happened to me. I feel very, very good about myself. I understand that it is not vain to want to be put together again.

How did your family react to your mastectomy and subsequent reconstruction?

My sons were 15 and 8 at the time. The 15-year-old was mature enough to hear about it. We discussed breast cancer and the possibility of a mastectomy. I told him that I was going into the hospital for a biopsy, and he asked what adults would not ask. He asked, "Are you going to die?" I said, "Jimmy, I sure hope not. I don't think so. That is what a mastectomy is all about." He went up to his room and was gone for a long time. I didn't really know what to do, whether to go talk to him or to leave him alone. I decided to leave him alone. He came to me later and said, "You're very lucky." I said, "Do you think so?" He said, "Absolutely. You told me you are not going to have any more babies and you don't need them for anything else anyway. It could have been inside, and they couldn't have done anything about it. On the outside, they can take it off and you can be okay." He got my perspectives in order fast. I approached the 8-year-old differently. I still told him about the surgery, but I was not as specific as I was with the 15-year-old.

My mother really surprised me with her reaction to my decision to get my breast reconstructed. I thought she would say, "Why do you want to do that?" Instead, she said, "I think you should do this thing." I didn't go into a lot of detail with my father; I didn't want to worry him. He had worried so much about my cancer surgery. I told him that my surgery was just for my vanity, and it was really no big deal. Fortunately, my parents were living out of state so they would not have to come every day and see me recuperating."

Was your husband supportive of you during your surgeries?

When I woke up from my mastectomy, my husband said, "Well, I was always a leg man anyway." He teased me immediately. We laughed the minute I woke up from surgery. We still laugh. There are people who are not lucky enough to have a sense of humor or somebody to share that humor with.

My husband really left the decision for reconstructive surgery up to me. He felt that I was the one who would have to experience the surgery, pain, and recuperation, so I would have to make the decision. If I wanted it, he would say, "Fine, terrific. Let's see what we can do." He went to his company to see if they could help us finance it. He really was wonderful.

What type of reconstructive procedure did you select?

I had a flap reconstruction. They took the latissimus dorsi back muscle and used it to build a breast mound and to fill out my hollowed chest. It was done in two stages or operations. This was the best procedure for me, because my normal breast was large and by using a flap, I had enough tissue to have my reconstructed breast match my remaining breast and still give me the filling out that I needed for the rest of my deformity.

Was your reconstructive surgery painful and how long did it take you to recuperate?

It took a good 6 or 7 weeks to recover and my mastectomy required only 5 or 6 weeks. I had more discomfort and pain with reconstruction than I did with my mastectomy. If a friend of mine were considering reconstruction, I would tell her about the 6-week recovery period. I would also tell her that compared to a lifetime of being reconstructed, 6 weeks is a small thing. Not every reconstruction is as involved as mine was. Usually your reconstruction parallels your original surgery. If it took a while to recover from the mastectomy, plan on the same type of recuperative period for the reconstruction.

Did you choose to have your nipple-areola reconstructed and why?

Yes, I did, but it was very much like pulling teeth to get me to go through with this last stage. I was sick of surgery and didn't know if I could face anymore. I didn't want to be sore again, and I was turned off by the fact that the skin for the areola is removed from the groin area and it smarts a lot. It's funny, but I thought I would be happy without a nipple, because all I really wanted was a breast shape and filling for the concave area under my breast. I thought the nipple really wasn't that important, but it is incredible how beautiful it is. It really is something. I am glad that I did it because now my breast is a finished product.

Did you have any surgery on your remaining breast?

Yes, I had the other side lifted and that was for symmetry, to make my breasts even.

Are you satisfied with the physical appearance of your reconstructed breast?

Yes, I am 100% happy with the size, match, balance, and cleavage of my breasts. If I have any complaint, it is with the firmness of the implant. When you lie down, one breast is up and one is down. That's it, though, and that is such a minor complaint compared to my overall pleasure at my aesthetic result.

There also isn't much that could be done about my scars. I have a diagonal scar that runs from the outermost part of my shoulder down almost to my waistline, and that scar will always be there. After 3 years, it faded pretty well. With reconstruction, the scar was reopened, however, and it has taken another 2 years to fade again. But, it is still there. I also have a tremendously long scar across my back from the latissimus dorsi reconstruction. This scar is very visible in a low-cut bathing suit. You need to be able to deal with these scars.

Does your reconstructive surgery limit your physical activity in any way?

There is a certain tightness in my shoulder and arm. I don't have quite the reach that I had before. I also have some feelings of limitation from tightness in my shoulder.

Did you require any therapy or exercise program after your reconstruction?

Yes, just moderate exercise moving the shoulder area. Basically, I did the same exercise that I used after my mastectomy.

How did you pay for your reconstruction and was it covered by insurance?

The story of how I paid for my reconstruction is an encouraging one. It gives you some idea of how corporations can be supportive of their employees. My husband had worked for one company when I had my mastectomy, but 3 years later, when I was discussing reconstruction, my husband had changed companies and reconstruction was not covered on the new policy. We found out that Blue Cross and Blue Shield would cover part of it, but that still left a big chunk of the expense not covered. My husband had gone through personnel to inquire about the insurance coverage, and the company agreed to underwrite anything that was not covered by the policy. So my reconstruction was fully paid for because his company stepped in and said: "Yes, we will be happy to pay for it."

If you had it to do over again, would you have your breast reconstructed immediately after your mastectomy surgery, so you would not have to experience breast loss?

This is an individual matter. I firmly believe that you need time between the mastectomy and the reconstruction. You have so much to deal with when you have a mastectomy. You are dealing with disfiguration, personal relationships, and cancer. You are healing physically; but there is so much to hear and think about psychologically that I wonder if you need to deal with reconstruction. I wonder if you would be as happy with it.

Maybe I am as happy as I am with my reconstructed breast because I had 3 years to totally come to grips with the idea of mastectomy and cancer. I had time to consider how I felt about myself and what direction I was going in. To be minus a breast for a while and deal with what you look like and then have reconstruction is wonderful. Consequently, when I had the reconstruction, I felt like it was this wonderful experience, like the frosting on the cake.

I might have been disappointed if I had reconstruction right away, before I knew what I would have looked like without a breast. Reconstructing a breast is not the same as giving someone back a natural breast. My plastic surgeon did the very best that he could do with the reconstruction. It is not a replacement, and it is not going to look the same. You are going to have a different feeling on that side. You are not going to have your natural feeling or your softness back. If you go to sleep, knowing that your breast is going to be removed, and then you wake up to find a reconstructed breast, I wonder if you can really be that happy with the reconstruction. I'm not too sure that you can. I'm not sure I needed 3 years between surgeries, but I definitely needed time between them.

How do people react when they learn that your breasts were reconstructed? Are women more sympathetic than men?

You would be amazed at how many people ask to see. I just tell them that it is my little hidden treasure, not really for their eyes. Most people stare at you; their eyes immediately go from your mouth to your chest to see what you look like. Many men react by questioning why you want to bother with it. The terror of surgery usually sobers them.

I have had some women tell me that they thought it was foolish. Interestingly enough, these women have had mastectomies themselves. Women who have never had mastectomies are usually very supportive. I think maybe if you have both of your breasts, you understand why somebody wants to come back to it, but if you have a mastectomy, sometimes reconstruction won't allow you to be a martyr anymore. That's probably why some women who have had mastectomies put it down. They don't realize some of their motivations, but the attention is important to them. I don't intend that in a mean way, but when you have had a mastectomy, people tell you that you are such a wonderful person and you are so brave and look at how well you have done. You would be surprised at the celebrity status it brings to a woman who hasn't had any attention. All of a sudden the world is at your door. People would say to me, "I could never have done it; you are so wonderful!" I couldn't relate to that. Of course they would have dealt with it. What else is there to do? It isn't as if you have an option.

When you choose to have your breast reconstructed, you take away some of that star status. You have a tendency to go on with your life and not reflect back. You feel and behave whole. You don't talk about it all the time. You don't tell people all the time, so you can get their reactions and hear, "You're such a wonderful person."

What advice would you like to give to other women considering breast reconstruction?

I think they have to ask themselves why they really want it and be more honest than I was with myself. I don't think they need to rationalize to get it.

It really matters what is happening in your life at the time of your mastectomy; this affects how you will cope and your need or desire for reconstruction. It matters if you are married. It matters if you are having a good relationship at the time you have a mastectomy. It matters if you are young, and if you have never been married. It matters if you are 60 years old and you are a widow. You still have a life ahead of you, and you don't know what the future holds or if you will ever have another personal relationship unless you can deal with it. And it infuriates me when everyone is lumped together in order to explain them or their actions. We are individuals with separate needs.

If a woman decides on breast reconstruction, she should definitely see more than one plastic surgeon and get more than one opinion. She should understand what kind of original surgery she has had, so she knows the extent of her deformity. If you have had a modified radical mastectomy, you are not going to have as big a deformity or as big an operation for reconstruction as you would if you had a radical mastectomy. Also, a woman has to ask herself if her age is going to make it difficult for her. Some women are considering reconstruction after 10 or 15 years. They need to ask what results they can expect. It is important for them to understand their results and for the doctor to be honest about what he hopes to accomplish. Nobody looks just like before, but you still look very nice.

It is important for people to stop seeing reconstruction as cosmetic and vain. "Oh, that woman is so vain because she went through all that." And they compare it to a facelift or a tummy tuck, and it is not the same thing at all. Psychologically, it does wonderful things.

CAROL: I COULDN'T WAIT

When Carol knocked on my hotel door, I was surprised to see how young she was. Slender, with dark, wavy hair, Carol is only 27 years old, and yet she has survived two breast cancers and the additional trauma of witnessing the development of cancer in other family members. Carol's grandmother, father, brother, and now sister have all been stricken by this disease. Still, she maintains a positive attitude about her life and her future.

Carol was only 21 and single when her first breast cancer was discovered. She still regrets her negligence in reporting her breast lump to her doctor, believing that early detection might have helped her more. Even so, her cancer was discovered in its early stages, before it had spread beyond local breast tissue. To treat her cancer, and on the recommendation of her general surgeon, Carol had a modified radical mastectomy followed by an immediate breast reconstruction with implant placement. Two years later, when another breast cancer was detected in her remaining breast, she made a conscious choice to repeat her initial therapy and again had an immediate breast reconstruction after her mastectomy.

The results of both of her immediate breast procedures were disappointing to Carol. Her breasts did not match and they were not what she expected. She experienced periods of depression over her appearance and worried how her "less than perfect breasts" would be perceived by the men in her life. "I expected my new breasts to be duplicates of what I had lost, and that just is not possible. It was probably immaturity on my part, because I never asked what they would look like. I just wanted to get it over with. I didn't want to hear anything bad. I wanted everything to be all right and positive." Carol has since undergone additional reconstructive procedures to enlarge her breasts and improve their contour and symmetry.

Despite her initial displeasure with the appearance of her reconstructed breasts, Carol strongly advocates having this surgery performed at the time of the mastectomy. She did not want to experience breast loss, and even when she was due for her first biopsy, she refused to sign any paper that would permit the surgeon to remove her breast. She definitely wanted her breasts intact when she wakened from her anesthesia. "I would have had a nervous breakdown if someone had told me that at 21 I would go into the hospital and come out with a flat chest. I was young, I was dating, and I just couldn't have handled it."

Carol admits that if you expect perfection, you probably will be dissatisfied with the results of immediate reconstruction, but that disappointment is minimal compared to the distress you feel when your breast is totally gone. Even though Carol had two immediate breast reconstructions, she did experience a brief period of breast loss when, after her second reconstruction, one of her implants had to be removed for 6 months to allow her tissues to heal more effectively. This experience was particularly devastating for her because it occurred right before her wedding, and she couldn't take pleasure in the nightgowns and pretty lingerie that she had been purchasing for her honeymoon.

Today, Carol is pleased with the final results of her reconstructed breasts, but it has taken almost 5 years, and several return visits to the operating room, for her to reach this level of satisfaction. Recently, her sister also developed breast cancer and had both breasts removed and immediately reconstructed. Now Carol is trying to help her adjust to a less than perfect result by reminding her that it will improve with time and further surgery. Carol realizes that even though an immediate reconstruction reduces the emotional trauma of mastectomy, a woman requires support and encouragement from her loved ones to help her adjust to the results of her surgery. Acknowledging the limitations of immediate surgery, she still feels that, for some patients, it is ultimately worthwhile. "I was a perfectionist; not every woman is that way. Some are happy to just have something there and don't want to come back for additional surgery to make their breasts look more normal. They probably just want to forget the whole experience. I felt a little like that, but I still wanted the best, and that is why I was willing to have my plastic surgeon operate on my breasts until they really looked good, nipples and all. It took a long time, but I kept my breasts, and with all of its imperfections, immediate breast reconstruction was the best approach for me."

How did you discover your breast cancer?

I first felt the lump as I was showering. At the time, it scared me but I didn't tell anyone about it. I waited, and then it swelled and I started to worry. Still, I kept quiet. I only went to the gynecologist because I had developed another problem that I could not ignore. If the doctor hadn't found my lump, I probably would never have told him about it. I was too scared. Now I tell everyone I know that if they find a breast lump, they should go see their doctors right away. I can't help thinking that if I had gone when I first found it, it might not have been as bad.

When my doctor discovered my lump, he sent me to a general surgeon for a breast biopsy. He assured me that my lump probably wasn't anything, but they would biopsy it to make sure. I felt that I was too young to have cancer and I wasn't really frightened, even though everybody else was. The biopsy didn't scare me, but I was terrified about the possibility of having to sign a paper—if cancer were discovered—allowing the surgeon to remove my breast while I was asleep. I did not want to wake up with nothing. I swore that I would never sign that paper. I didn't need to, however, because the results of the biopsy were negative and I was allowed to go home.

The next week, the doctor called and told me to bring my mother in with me for a consultation. I started to worry, even though I never asked him why he wanted to see us. I don't like to hear bad news, and I've found that if I don't ask, I don't get upset. During our visit, the doctor explained that the lump hadn't looked right to him, and despite the negative frozen-section diagnosis, he sent a sample of the lump to a laboratory in Utah for further testing. This time it came out positive for cancer. Luckily, the cancer had just started.

Why did you decide to have your breasts reconstructed immediately after your mastectomies?

You have to remember that I was very young when all of this was first happening. The surgeon really told us what he thought was the best thing to do. He talked more to my mom than he did to me, and I just sat there and said, "Oh, God, What now?" Our doctor was very reassuring and said, "We are going to perform a mastectomy, and then a plastic surgeon will rebuild your breast." I didn't really make a decision; I just followed, but I wouldn't have wanted it to be any other way. They had already set a date for surgery and reserved a hospital room, and everything was ready to go. We met with the doctor on Thursday, and I went into the hospital on the next Monday. Fortunately, I didn't have much time to dwell on what was happening to me.

Just having the doctor say, "We're going to build you one." did it for me. If he had said, "We're going to take your breast off," I think I would have fallen apart. I would have died. I was young and I was dating, and my breasts were important to me, they still are, but he gave me hope. I thought, "He is going to take off my real breast, but I am going to wake up with a new, beautiful one."

When my second breast cancer was discovered in my remaining breast, I handled it better, knowing that I could have an immediate reconstruction. I asked the surgeon, "Well, are you going to do what you did the last time with the plastic surgeon?" and when he said "yes," I was pleased.

Was your reconstructive surgery painful and how long did it take you to recuperate?

It was very painful. Every muscle in your chest is pulled, and it hurts to get up. I think it hurts so much because you are recovering from two surgeries, a mastectomy and a breast reconstruction, at the same time. You can't lift anything. You can walk, but it is very slow. It takes over a week to get over that, and it took me a good month or two before I felt that I was back to normal, or before I could lift anything heavy. You also can't raise your arms at the beginning.

Every time I went in to have my implant changed, I had to stay in the hospital overnight, and I didn't feel good for 4 to 5 days afterward.

Does your reconstructive surgery limit your physical activity in any way?

No, not really. I can do most ordinary activities. I have to be a little more careful when I'm involved in sports. I ski, and my plastic surgeon told me to make sure that I fall on my back and not my front, because I could move my implant out of place. Wouldn't that be something? Can't you picture me coming down the slope with my boob moved around to my back? I try to think humorously about it, but I probably could push it out of place if I weren't careful. He's never cautioned me about waterskiing. I also exercise regularly and that is no problem. After surgery, I couldn't exercise for about 3 weeks, but now I can do almost anything that I want to do.

Were you pleased with the physical results of your immediate breast reconstructions?

I always had it in my mind that I was going to be beautiful after surgery. I didn't ask any questions. If they had told me in the beginning that my breasts would not have looked perfect, that might have ruined it for me. I did not realize that it was going to be a long process of rebuilding my breasts and might take me 4 or 5 years to make them look normal.

I went into surgery with two normal-appearing breasts, and I woke up with a reconstructed breast that didn't look perfect. My plastic surgeon kept saying, "Oh, this is beautiful," but I thought he was sick. It didn't look like I thought it would look; it didn't look normal. I didn't cry or think that I was ugly and would never get married; those thoughts never entered my mind. I just felt sad.

They never told me that my breasts wouldn't look the same after surgery. They never told me that my breasts would be scarred and numb, and I never asked. When I discovered that I had no sensitivity or feeling in my breasts, all I could think about was being out with a guy who had wandering hands, and me not even knowing what he was doing.

For a while, it seemed as if I were having operations almost every 6 months to build my breast and make it symmetrical with the remaining, normal one. After my second breast reconstruction, my plastic surgeon worked on both breasts at the same time. With every operation, my plastic surgeon said, "I'm going to make you a little bigger." And I thought, "Oh, good," but every time I was disappointed. They were never big enough, and I wanted them to be perfect, and they are never going to be perfect. I guess that is where the immaturity comes in. Truthfully, it has taken me from the time I was 21 until I was 26 to be happy with them. Still, I am not totally satisfied with my scars, and my nipples poke out all the time, almost as if they were cold. Sometimes, I put Band-Aids over them so they won't show through my shirt.

I used to get upset, because I wanted my breasts to be the same size. My mom would say, "Carol, my breasts aren't the same size." But when you don't have your real breasts anymore, you don't remember whether yours were the same size or not. You want them to look normal or what you remember as normal. My Mom would say, "Carol, look at mine. See, they are different." Still, it wasn't the same. I'm more satisfied now.

When you discovered that your reconstructed breasts were not what you had expected, did you encounter any problems in dating or forming intimate relationships?

I had been engaged to someone, and when we broke up, I worried, "How am I going to have relationships with anyone in this condition?" Not long after, I started dating someone else, but I would not take off my shirt when we went to bed. I kept it on for a long time. I dated him for 2 years, and he helped me. When he first saw my breasts, he told me how pretty he thought they were. I think that he was just amazed at what surgery could accomplish.

When I started dating the man who became my husband, my shirt went back on. I guess that is natural. I have scars, and I was afraid that a man would want to know about them. A man plays a big part in helping a woman adjust to her body. If it weren't for those two, if they hadn't encouraged me and worked with me, I would have had a much more difficult time adjusting. It's nice to know that you are accepted, admired, and regarded as attractive by someone of the opposite sex.

What problems or complications did you have with your breast reconstructions?

I didn't have any with the first reconstruction, but with the second, my implant had to be removed. I was supposed to relax and recuperate. But, that's hard for me to do. I'm an impatient person. If I want something done, I don't want to wait. I want it done immediately. If I were lying in bed and I saw a cobweb, it would drive me crazy until I removed it. I did everything that I was not supposed to do. If the dishes needed washing, I would wash them. My scar kept splitting open. My plastic surgeon put some tape on it and told me not to do anything more, but again I did not listen and it did not heal properly. Finally, he had to remove my implant, and that was painful.

When your implant was removed, did you feel as if you had experienced a mastectomy?

Yes, even though I originally had two immediate breast reconstructions, I went without a breast for 6 months, and it happened at the worst time for me. I was going to be married, and I only had one breast for my wedding; that was truly depressing. My weakness is gowns; I love beautiful, flowing, sexy gowns, and I was getting so many wonderful ones for my wedding, but I couldn't wear them. I just cried and cried. It never bothered Jim (my husband), just me.

During this 6 months, I had to wear this thing that the American Cancer Society gave me, a little cotton form. Oh Lord, if I had to wear that the rest of my life I would die. I hated it. And you can't wear gowns. It was summer, and I had to stick it inside my bathing suit when I went swimming. My mom would sew it in, but it still did not look the same, and I was always worrying that it would float out in the water. After that experience, I'd have reconstructions every 6 months for the rest of my life just to always have breasts, rather than having nothing.

If your original mastectomies and reconstructions were so painful, why have you submitted to additional elective surgery?

After every operation, I think that I will never go through this again. It hurts too much and I just won't do it again. But then, after a little while, I reconsider if surgery will make my breasts look better. If my plastic surgeon came in today and said that he wanted to operate again next week to make them more symmetrical, I'd say okay.

How did your family react to your mastectomy and reconstruction?

My mom was always there for me. It would have been very difficult for me without her help, just being there handing me water or doing my chores.

We have had so much cancer in our family that she goes crazy every time she thinks of it. I try not to do that; I don't cry. I take things out on my mom because she tries to baby me. I fight it. She cries all of the time. You tend to run away from all of that; you don't want to encounter it. I don't blame her; she had been through so much. Since I've experienced it with my younger sister, I can see what my mom has suffered, and I wish I hadn't treated her so hatefully some of the times.

How has your husband reacted to all of your surgery?

Generally, Jim has been very supportive. He keeps telling me that he is a rear man anyway, and he doesn't really care about breasts. Still, he always tells me that my breasts look just fine to him. It hurts him that I have to have them operated on, but he tries not to make an issue of it. Right now, he is tired of all of my reconstructive surgery. He has told me that he does not want me to go back for any more, because it is painful and I am confined to bed. He worries about me. As far as I am concerned, and we have discussed my feelings, I will continue to have more surgery as long as it makes me feel better or as long as I feel it is necessary. I know that he understands my position, even though he is not totally happy with it.

How can men be supportive of women who have had mastectomies and breast reconstruction?

My husband has been wonderful. For a long time I wore a shirt to bed, or I only took it off in the dark, but he was patient with me until I reached a point where I didn't feel self-conscious. He tells me that I look great.

I realize how important a man's support is, when I see what my sister is currently experiencing. She just had both of her breasts removed and immediately reconstructed. Her husband makes her feel terrible. Joan, like me, did not have perfect results with her immediate surgery, but she should have known what to expect after having seen what I went through. I guess each person has to experience it for herself. The difference is that I have a loving, supportive husband, and I still feel good about myself. I think my sister would feel better if her husband were more supportive. Recently, she came to me crying and asked if my husband had ever told me to put my shirt back on. Of course, I said, "No." Then she told me that her husband looked at her the previous evening, as she was undressing, and told her to put her shirt back on and turn around. She probably shouldn't tell me things like that; it just irritates me.

My sister has been seeing a psychiatrist to help her adjust, and I think it is a good idea. But even a psychiatrist can't help you, if your husband doesn't help. Her doctor suggested that she ask her husband what he likes best about her and then every time that she thought about her breasts she should instead focus on what he liked best. Well, she tried that, and her husband couldn't think of anything. He said that he was going to have to think about it, and he has yet to tell her. That does something to you. She told me, "What am I, Carol? Am I ugly? What is wrong with me? Are my breasts the only thing he thinks of?" I told her to leave him, but she won't because she thinks that nobody else will ever want her. No matter how strong your self-image is, you are definitely influenced by how men regard and treat you.

Did your insurance cover the cost of your initial reconstructions and your subsequent surgeries?

I had some problems with my last surgery. The insurance company said that it was cosmetic, because the plastic surgeon made my breasts larger. Anyone knowing anything about me or my surgery, knew how ridiculous that was, but the insurance company was insistent. It got to be over a year and they still had not paid, and I could not get them to do anything, so I called my mom's lawyer, and he filed a claim and they paid.

Are you satisfied with your breasts now?

Yes. They are even and they look much better. It is wonderful being able to wear all types of clothing again. I like wearing bras, sundresses, and sexy nightgowns. When my plastic surgeon got my breasts to the point where I was satisfied with them, I went out and bought the prettiest nightgown that I could find and I wore it that night. It fit me. For years, I haven't had anything that really fit me like that. I was the happiest person in the world. I feel very good about my appearance now.

If you had it to do over again, would you have your breasts reconstructed immediately, at the time of your mastectomy, or after a delay, which might allow you to have an improved result with less additional surgery?

I would do it again in the exact same way. Immediate reconstruction just makes you feel better, despite any imperfections. You know that after surgery you will have something there and you are not going to wake up without your breast.

DIANE: THE STIGMA IS GONE

Diane is a vivacious, red-headed woman with a youthful appearance and a trim figure. During our interview,* I was surprised to learn that she is over 50 and has three grown children. Her manner was warm and intimate, and she spoke to me without restraint about her experiences with mastectomy and reconstruction.

Three years ago, Diane had a radical mastectomy followed by a year of chemotherapy as a precaution because she had positive lymph nodes. Her mastectomy was devastating for her and she labeled herself as seriously "deformed." She had a hollow arm and chest, a long scar, and no breast. She hated to even look at herself in the mirror. When she heard about the possibility of having her breast reconstructed, Diane was overjoyed. "It gave me something to look forward to. When I was taking chemotherapy, it helped me to know that down the road I had an option if I wanted it." Even the loss of her thick, red hair during chemotherapy didn't bother her, because she knew that not only would her hair grow back, but she also could restore her breast through breast reconstruction.

Two years later, Diane's breast was reconstructed with a latissimus dorsi (back muscle) flap. Her breast mound was restored and her hollow arm and chest area were filled in. In addition, her axillary fold (armpit area) was restored. To achieve symmetry, her remaining breast was augmented by placing a silicone implant under the muscle. Diane's reconstructive surgery produced physical and psychological benefits. "There was a change in my personality the day after I got home from the hospital. I felt whole again, and, gee that was great! Every facet of my life changed."

Diane is now involved in directing her local Reach to Recovery chapter, a nonprofit organization dedicated to helping other women who have had mastectomies for breast cancer and to getting them

---

*An interview with Diane's husband Bill is included in Chapter 14.

back into the mainstream of life. Diane's husband also has become involved in this effort; he talks to the husbands and boyfriends of women with mastectomies and offers them encouragement and assistance. As Diane and I talked, she told me of a recent conversation that she had with a young patient in a mental health outpatient facility. After a mastectomy this woman had totally withdrawn from the world, refusing to bathe, dress, or even remove her clothes. The hospital nurse had asked Diane to see if she could help this patient to realize that other women had encountered some of the same experiences. Diane shared her own chemotherapy memories, including the loss of her hair and the necessity for buying a wig. Throughout her conversation, Diane was sadly aware of "this poor girl's inability to cope with her cancer or her mastectomy. Mastectomy had destroyed her self-image and psychologically devastated her." Reflecting further on her own personal experiences with mastectomy and the happiness that she has experienced by having breast reconstruction, Diane felt that this alternative was a very positive means of psychological rehabilitation and that information about its benefits should be shared with other women.

What are the benefits of reconstruction?

To me the biggest benefit of reconstruction is that it removes the stigma of cancer. After my mastectomy, I just didn't feel whole. It is hard to explain. Even though I looked okay when dressed with my prosthesis, I knew the difference. You have to feel good inside to look pretty outside.

Taking a bath and getting dressed in the mornings and evenings was the worst thing for me to cope with. When I would look at myself in the bathroom mirror, and there is a lot of mirror in the bathroom (I threatened to break it, but I didn't), I would see myself and immediately think of cancer. It is just there. You are branded.

I would always dress and undress in the bathroom, because I didn't want my husband to see me. That was my biggest concern; that was my stigma. To get rid of that feeling is terrific, because now I look at myself and I'm happy and I don't think cancer. I look and I say, "Oh, you beautiful thing." I don't care if he sees me or not. For the best testimony to breast reconstruction, you should really be talking to my husband. He says there is a big difference in my personality from the time I had cancer to after reconstruction. Even my relationship with my husband has changed; I enjoy sex more. He tells my friends that it's hard to keep my clothes on now. He is so pleased. The kids are gone, and I think, "Gee whiz, it's fun to run around." But life is so much fun now compared to before. I am back like I was. In fact, I'm better because he enlarged my other breast, and I can wear clothes without a bra. I had three kids, and now I look great.

Breast reconstruction meant an extra plus in my life at an age (my fifties) when you weigh those decisions. I determined that age didn't have anything to do with whether or not I had surgery. If I can enjoy this through my remaining years, great. In fact, if I had died within a year or two, the surgery would still have been worth it; it really would. It is wonderful to be able to go out there and shop and buy pretty lingerie. Things like that really appeal to me again.

Was your reconstructive surgery painful and would you do it again?

Yes, I would do it again. This surgery is a happy experience. I really didn't have much pain. We're all different, with varying degrees of pain. I think you can pretty much gauge your pain level for reconstruction by comparing it with your pain experience during your mastectomy. I didn't have a bad time with either operation, and my recuperation time was short. I was up and about when I got home, even though I couldn't drive or lift for a few weeks. I could go out to dinner right away. I really wasn't handicapped.

Were you prepared for the results of your reconstruction?

Well, you visualize the way you are going to look and then you are a little afraid to check and see how you really look. I'll never forget the day they came in to check me, and the young doctor and the nurse unwrapped me. I was sitting up in bed and feeling like an oddity, but I wouldn't look. The second day I looked down at my real breast, which had been augmented, and oh it looked so big. And I said, "Oh my goodness, you beautiful thing." I thought it was so gorgeous that I called my neighbor and said, "You wouldn't believe what a beautiful boob I have." Then, when I saw my other one, my reconstructed one, I told my sister, "You've got to come up here and see my new boob." It was so much fun. I shared it with all my family, because I think you should.

Are you satisfied with the results of your reconstruction?

Yes, my breasts are just beautiful. The reconstructed breast is very soft, my cleavage is good, and so is my breast contour. The reconstructed breast is a little darker than my normal breast and I have very little sexual sensitivity in my reconstructed breast, but I think these are minor items. My scar is still red, but it will fade.

Did you choose to have your nipple-areola reconstructed and why?

Yes, I wanted it to be finished. That is all part of being a woman because of that little plus and it just added that much. I just wanted it all to be there.

How do people react when they learn that your breasts were reconstructed?

Their eyes drop; sometimes it's fun to wear a tight sweater. People notice the change in you. They say, "You feel good." and I say "Yes, and I'm happy." Some people don't understand why I had more surgery; they view the operation as more pain and don't understand the psychological implications. I guess being older has helped me to handle some of the questions and doubts. I'm at an age where once I made my decision that reconstruction was right for me and I was going to do it, I was able to cope with it.

What used to kill me is when a person would say to me, "Gee, you look fine to me. Why do you want reconstruction?" What I wanted to say was "Hey, you should be around when I'm taking my bath; you'd run like a turkey." They meant well, but their comments still hurt.

How can people be more sensitive to cancer and reconstruction patients?

People talk so much without thinking. For instance, when you are going through chemotherapy, you don't feel terrific but you muster enough energy to carry on. Then some people will approach you and say, "Oh my goodness, you don't look sick. You mean you're on chemotherapy?" and go on and on. They should keep their mouths shut.

Another bothersome habit is when a friend or family member comes and tells you about Aunt Martha. She lost both breasts; how lucky you are that you lost one. Or Aunt Suzy died and this just goes on all the time. I want to say, "Listen, it's me, not Aunt Martha. I know I'm lucky, but I don't like to be told. All I need to know is that you care." Also, when you visit in the hospital, don't worry about what to say; don't say anything. Let the patient talk; be a good listener.

How can a man be supportive in decisions concerning breast cancer and breast reconstruction?

My husband has been very supportive, but he really didn't encourage me to have the breast reconstruction because he hated to see me go through more surgery after a year of chemotherapy. He said, "Don't you think you have had enough?" But he also said, "It has to be your decision." He wanted me to understand that I was not doing it for him, but I had to be doing it for myself. He said, "If you want it for you I'll go along with it." From that point on he was with me every step of the way.

BETTY: I WANT IT FOR ME

A slender, feminine woman in her midforties, Betty appeared uncomfortable as she was introduced to me at our interview. She later confided that she wasn't sure that she knew what to say to me. Fortunately for both of us, Betty had much to share, and she gave me new insights into how some women cope with breast cancer.

Coping for Betty meant putting on a brave front and getting on with her life. Although she obviously had deep feelings about her cancer experience, Betty was reluctant to display them. When her surgeon first told her that she had breast cancer, instead of crying or bemoaning what had befallen her, Betty reacted by saying, "OK, let's get it over with. Get it out of me; I don't need it." Even after her mastectomy, Betty did not outwardly allow herself a period of grieving, but immediately sought information about her rehabilitation. When her surgeon told her about the possibility of reconstructive breast surgery, Betty enthusiastically embraced this option and decided that if she were a candidate, she would like to have this operation. She "didn't want to bother with a prosthesis" and reconstructive surgery would be "perfect for her." She wanted it for "her self-image and so she could wear pretty clothes and put the cancer experience behind her." Four weeks after her mastectomy, Betty called a plastic surgeon to set up an appointment to discuss reconstructive surgery. Her mastectomy surgery was in April 1981. In September 1981 she had her breast reconstruction, and in January 1982 she had her nipple-areola reconstructed. Betty did not allow herself a long convalescence and was up and around within 5 days after her reconstructive surgery.

Because Betty had a modified radical mastectomy with her chest wall muscles preserved, her plastic surgeon was able to reconstruct her breast by inserting an implant under her muscle and using the available tissue left from her mastectomy. In addition to reconstruction, her remaining breast was modified to match her reconstructed breast; it was reduced and uplifted. Her surgery was performed in two procedures, the first under general anesthesia and the nipple reconstruction under local anesthesia. Betty had the simplest form of reconstruction and was thrilled with her results. Of all the women that I interviewed, Betty is the one who enthusiastically opened her dress to reveal her reconstructed breast and show me how her scar had miraculously faded.

Today, Betty is confronting another crisis because she and her husband have recently been divorced. Even though she admits that sometimes she feels depressed, she still believes that breast reconstruction represents a "plus in her life" and has helped her to cope with some of her current problems.

Why did you seek reconstruction?

I wanted reconstruction for my self-image. I wanted to wear pretty bras, and I didn't want to be bothered with a prosthesis. Right after my mastectomy, my husband and I went to the Far East and I was wearing my prosthesis. I just didn't feel that fantastic in my clothes, and I have some beautiful clothes. That night I wore a long black dress and during the evening the prosthesis slipped and I thought, "I just cannot wait for reconstruction so I can wear fancy things and be comfortable again."

I think reconstruction is the most marvelous thing that can happen to a woman after mastectomy. If you have to have a mastectomy, get it over with and then—if you want it—you can be reconstructed. But you must want it and you don't want to do it for someone else. It makes you feel like a whole woman. I didn't feel like a half woman, necessarily, when I had the mastectomy, but I thought that if I could get one back why not go for it.

How did your family react to your mastectomy and subsequent breast reconstruction?

My husband told me, "This will not affect the way I feel about you." He was marvelous at the time. Of course now I am beginning to think a little differently about how he felt because we are divorced. Back then he was wonderful. In fact, he was so wonderful he drove me crazy. He would come in with a cup of coffee and a paper and sit and sit. Finally, I just threw him out of the hospital. "Go play golf," I said. "Let me get up, do my exercises, and have some fun with the other patients. Get out of here."

Now, my daughter was very much afraid. She wasn't afraid for me necessarily, but I could just see fear in her eyes. I told her, "Honey, I'm still your mom; it's still me." Then I asked her if she were afraid for herself and she said, "Yes." I made sure that she had herself checked. Then everything was okay.

Both my husband and daughter were happy about my decision to have breast reconstruction. They were very supportive.

How can a man be more supportive to a woman going through these experiences?

He needs to stroke. He still needs to touch, and that means more than saying, "I love you and this surgery is not going to bother me." Women need hugs and caresses; it makes you feel special and cared about.

Was your reconstructive surgery painful and how long did it take you to recuperate?

I am pretty good with pain. The pain from the mastectomy was not that great; the worst part was when they pulled the drain out and took off the adhesive tape. Adhesive tape sticks and blisters and I'm allergic to it. Right before I was to have my reconstruction, I told my plastic surgeon that I did not want any adhesive tape. I was almost under the anesthetic. "What do you mean you don't want any adhesive tape?" he said. "What are we going to do?" I said, "I don't care what you do, but I don't want any adhesive tape because I'm allergic to it." So they wrapped me in elastic bandages. It was marvelous.

I can tolerate pain. The reconstruction was even easier than the mastectomy. I went up for surgery at 6 AM and at 10 AM I was telling them to take the IV out of my arm because I was hungry and I wanted to eat. When my plastic surgeon came in at 11:30 that morning he said, "They told me that you were sitting up and wanting food. I didn't believe them, but there you are." I was out of the hospital in 4 to 5 days. With the nipple reconstruction I was out of there in 3 days, even though I could have left after 2 days. I had no pain. I took pain pills home with me, but they are still up in the closet.

Are you satisfied with the physical appearance of your reconstructed breast?

I am very pleased. My plastic surgeon used my original mastectomy incision for the reconstruction. He opened a small section and inserted the implant. My scars are almost completely faded, because he told me about taking vitamin E pills and putting vitamin E oil on the scars. It took about 6 weeks of using the oil before the scars started to fade. At first the scar was straight across so I could not wear strapless or low-cut dresses, but after awhile it faded and curved. Now I can wear dresses cut to the navel if I want, and you don't see the scar. It is just marvelous.

I am happy with my nipple reconstruction but I wish it were a little bit darker, because the nipple on my normal breast is darker, but you just do the best you can. I also have hair growing out of my nipple; it's from the thigh area. My surgeon told me that the hair means that my plastic surgeon got a really good skin graft when he made the areola.

I am very satisfied with the size, balance, softness, and cleavage of my breasts. By massaging my breasts and keeping active, I have helped keep them soft. I have very little sensitivity in the reconstructed breast. The skin is sensitive, but sexually it is not responsive.

Did you have any surgery on your remaining breast?

Yes, I had it reduced to match the remaining one and my nipple was moved up on my breast. My plastic surgeon said, "Betty, I am going to have you looking like you are 16." I love it.

Did you have any complications as a result of your surgery?

Yes, I had some fluid buildup and I had to have it drained twice, but it really didn't restrict my activities. I went to my twenty-fifth high school reunion the next weekend and felt fine.

Did you require any therapy or exercise programs after your breast reconstruction?

Yes, my surgeon asked me to move my reconstructed breast around for about 5 minutes twice a day to try to keep it as soft as possible.

Has reconstruction caused you to curtail or restrict any of your physical activities?

No, I played golf 2 months after my mastectomy. It hurt like hell when I swung the club, but it loosened the more I used it. Then I took ballet. Ballet has done more for my reaching than anything. It's great exercise.

How did you pay for your reconstruction and was it covered by insurance?

My insurance covered it because in our state it is not considered cosmetic surgery.

If you had it to do over again would you have your reconstruction immediately after your mastectomy surgery so you would not have to experience the loss of your breast?

I don't think so. I don't think it would have worked as well. I think the healing of the scar is better, especially in my case because it had some time to settle after the mastectomy. My skin was supple and pliable and there was no problem reopening a part of the incision and putting in the implant. No, I definitely wouldn't have wanted it immediately because you are already going through one trauma coping with cancer, and I don't think you need to confront two or three issues at one time. There is enough shock there with the cancer. What I would want, however, is for my plastic surgeon to be present at the operation if I had to have another mastectomy. I would want him to help in deciding where the scar will be and in closing the incision.

How has reconstruction affected your life?

I think it has made me a happier person. Right after my breast was reconstructed, people could notice the difference in me. I would just beam. At the moment, I am going through a personal crisis because of my divorce but the mastectomy doesn't have anything to do with that, and the reconstruction has actually helped me to deal with it.

What advice would you like to give other women considering breast reconstruction?

Tell the girls out there that the loss suffered from a mastectomy does not have to last. You can have reconstruction and you will look and feel like a woman. It has meant so much to me to have reconstruction and it has meant it to me and not to anybody else.

CINDY: I WANTED THE BEST

"When I realized that I was going to have a mastectomy, my surgeon told me that I could have reconstructive breast surgery in a year. That information was probably the most important to me at that point. I felt good knowing that after I went through with my mastectomy, there was something that they could do, and I was not always going to be deformed looking. Knowing in my mind that I was able to have my breasts restored was what really kept my sanity during that time."

These words were spoken to me during my interview with Cindy, a petite, 36-year-old mother of three who impressed me with the effort she had invested in educating herself about all aspects of breast reconstruction. She had realistic expectations for what this surgery could produce, and she took the time to find the best plastic surgeon to perform her breast reconstruction. Cindy wanted to be sure "that it was done right the first time." Then she actively participated in the planning of that surgery.

Cindy had four or five biopsies before one of her breast lumps was diagnosed as malignant. To treat her cancer, she had a modified radical mastectomy on her right breast and a prophylactic mastectomy (to prevent cancer) on her left breast. The prophylactic procedure was done to remove the breast tissue that, at biopsy, was shown to have early signs of disease. Cindy had no positive lymph nodes, and chemotherapy was not recommended. Even though Cindy felt deformed by her surgery, she was relieved that her cancer had been found before it had spread. Only a year earlier, one of her friends had died of breast cancer, leaving two small children behind. Thus, Cindy was grateful that she could have a favorable prognosis, and she was looking forward to restoring her breasts.

Cindy sought breast reconstruction 6 months after her mastectomies. Her breasts were reconstructed with latissimus dorsi flaps, and her nipples were reconstructed 2 months later. The procedure that she selected was more involved than the reconstruction with available tissues selected by Betty, but it had the advantage of providing extra tissue to create larger breasts for Cindy. "I said that as long as you are doing it, do it good. Give me a nice-sized, B cup. I figured as long as I was going to have this operation, I wanted the most for my money. I didn't want to be huge or out of proportion, but he did an excellent job for my size and that is what I wanted." Cindy's quest for the right plastic surgeon to perform this surgery was a part of her desire to "do the best she could with what she had." She was not willing to leave this choice to chance.

Why did you seek reconstruction?

I remember going home after my mastectomy, removing the bandages, and looking at myself; it was very difficult, really, really hard. Of course, I didn't dare let anybody else look at me. You know, you just don't. Somehow I just went on with life. I was consoled knowing that I could be with my kids, and I wasn't going to die and leave my kids without a mother.

Six weeks after my mastectomy, I went to be fitted for my prosthesis. They brought out all of these forms for me to try on and nothing looked good. I was so upset at trying to get them to look good and to find the right kind. There were at least ten different styles and they were all thrust upon me, and I just left. I was shaking all over, and I thought, "I have to get out of here." I didn't buy anything. I couldn't handle it at that moment. I was just getting adjusted to what I was having to wear anyway. It was too upsetting. So I didn't buy anything like that. I just continued to wear what I had. I bought some little, cheap forms at Penneys, because I was not going to invest $200 or $300 in a form if I could have the reconstruction done. Anyway, my insurance would only pay for either reconstructive surgery or a prosthesis; it would not pay for both.

Those cheap prostheses were weird; when I put them in I felt as if I were all foam rubber walking around. One day when I was sitting in a chair, my daughter came and sat down in my lap and one of them popped up and I thought, "Ooooh." Little incidents like that give you a pang. I just went ahead and suffered through it until I was able to have the reconstructive surgery done.

I'm so glad that I had my breasts restored. I feel great when I'm dressed. I'm not afraid that a pad is going to be sticking out or something is going to be showing. Before I had reconstruction, sometimes I would go out and have to check to make sure that my breasts were still straight. I would worry that one of my forms would be up and one would be down. I also wore fuller blouses so people would not look at me. I wore nothing tight that would emphasize my breasts. Now, I don't have to worry about being lopsided. Now I can buy T-shirts that I wore before my mastectomy.

I was determined to have my breasts reconstructed if I could because I wanted to feel like I was put back together again. It accomplished that. I am an outgoing person and I don't usually let things get me down, but that was important. It doesn't matter how strong or tough other people think you are, some things can really bother you and get to you. So if you can help yourself by getting reconstructive breast surgery to make you feel good again, I think you should do it.

How did you choose the plastic surgeon to reconstruct your breasts?

I was looking for somebody who could assure me that he knew what he was doing and that he had already done a lot of other reconstructions. I went to doctors who told me that they would have to do one side at a time, and they couldn't guarantee what my breasts would look like. I was in tears after I came home for the first few doctors I consulted. One of them said, "No, I can't guarantee what you are going to look like. We may be able to take the muscle from the back and move it around, but we can only do one side, and I don't know about the nipple. We may have to remove the other nipple. I don't think that we will be able to share."

When I visited all of these doctors, I was very upset by the fact that everybody took pictures of me. I know that they had to do it, but it is very difficult to stand up against the wall, with the nurse and doctor there, and then allow them to take pictures of you at all angles. Probably if it had happened once or twice, it wouldn't have been so bad, but by the time you have been through four or five doctors, you just feel awful. I think doctors need to know that women feel this way.

If I had let the first doctor I consulted do my breast reconstruction, there is no telling what I would have looked like. Once you have it done, that's it. What else can you do? That is why it was so important for me to feel like I had found the doctor who did more breast reconstruction than anything else and was the most qualified to do this surgery. I wanted to know that when I woke up I was going to look good or at least the best that I could look under the circumstances. I didn't expect to look the way I did before my mastectomies.

The plastic surgeon I chose to perform my reconstructive surgery seemed to know how I was feeling and how important it was for me to look good again. He allowed me to see examples of his results, both good and bad, and to talk to other women who had this surgery. He made me feel as if he were interested in me and saw me as an individual. After surgery, my doctor did not lose interest; he did not hesitate to say, "Gee, you really look great." Everything had to be just right, or he wasn't going to be satisfied.

***Was your reconstructive surgery painful and how long did it take you
to recuperate?***

> I have a pretty high pain level. After my mastectomy, I only stayed
> home from work 3 weeks. I had company the night I came home
> from the hospital, and they said, "I can't believe it; you don't look
> like you had anything done. You look okay." I guess when people
> hear that you had breast surgery for cancer, they think that they are
> going to come in and find you dying right there on your bed. For
> me, getting back into a normal routine was good, and I pushed my-
> self to do that. I had to get back out and prove to myself that I could
> keep going.
>
> What I remember most about my breast reconstruction was the
> nausea from being under the anesthesia so long. The pain was not
> that bad. I think that I was so thrilled at having my breasts restored
> that pain didn't concern me. They gave me a pain pill and that did
> it for me. My recuperation was pretty speedy. I went home after 5
> days and back to work after 3 weeks.

Why did you choose to have your nipple-areola reconstructed?

> Because you *could* have it done. Why wouldn't you want to finish
> the job? To me it was just completing a job that we had started. I
> didn't have any reservations about doing it.
>
> I had the nipple put on under local anesthesia. They put a little
> mushroom-looking dressing on top of it. When the dressing was
> taken off, I can remember laughing and telling my friends that I
> hesitated to take a shower because I was afraid it would wash down
> the drain.

Are you satisfied with the physical appearance of your reconstructed breasts?

> I'm perfectly satisfied with my results. The color is perfect. The soft-
> ness is good and so is the degree of balance and cleavage. My breasts
> have no sensitivity, but they look good. My scars are still red, but
> they are fading. The scar on my back is hidden by my bra, but I
> have some blouses that have fuller armholes, and I cannot wear
> them because the scars would show. There is certain clothing that
> you cannot wear, but you accept it and wear something else. What is
> important is that I feel better about myself and I look more feminine
> and sexually attractive.
>
> I had realistic expectations going into breast reconstruction. I had
> no visions of grandeur; I knew that I was still going to be scarred. I
> knew that the nipple was not going to be exactly like the other nip-

ple. What I wanted was a plastic surgeon who would do the best with what he had to work with. That is why I am so satisfied, because in my mind I feel that I got the best job possible, and so I have no complaints about it.

Were you restricted in your physical activities after reconstructive surgery?

No. I went home, I ran, played tennis, played volleyball, and everything. There are times when you are going to be sore, but you just accept that as part of it. You can't have surgery and not expect some discomfort.

Are there any limitations or problems with your reconstructed breasts?

I still have a little pain. Sometimes, when I am lying on my back at night, I want to hold my breast forward because it still wants to fall back and to the side more than I like. So when I lie down, I find myself crossing my arms in order to pull my breasts to the front. My breasts are also numb. I don't have any normal feeling there or under my arms when I shave; it is still a very dead feeling. Shaving under your arm is a terrible feeling. At first, it almost nauseates you. It has taken me a long time to adjust to this numbness. I guess you eventually forget about it and go on. What can I say? That is a very, very minor complaint. I am just thankful that everything worked out and that I could have it done. Even my scars don't bother me; in fact they are already beginning to fade.

How did you pay for your breast reconstruction and was it covered by insurance?

It was covered by insurance, but my policy provided that they would pay for a prosthesis *or* breast reconstruction; they would not cover both. I also had to have the reconstructive surgery done within 1 year or I would not have 100% coverage.

If you had to do it again, would you like to have your breasts reconstructed immediately after your mastectomy?

No, I don't think I would want to have it done right away. Psychologically, you are going through enough with the mastectomy. First, I wanted to make sure that I was going to be okay and that the tissue was going to soften. I took one step at a time. I was willing to take whatever time was necessary to make each step successful.

I have a friend who had her breast reconstructed at the time she had her mastectomy. Since then she has had nothing but trouble.

She was unhappy about the work that had been done. Originally she felt she just had to have it done right away so that nobody would ever see her looking that way. That was important to her, but now she is unhappy with the results. I felt and still feel that this surgery is important enough to have it done right. The short delay was worth it, because my reconstructed breasts will be with me forever.

Was reconstructive surgery worth the time, pain, and money?

Yes, because what is 1 or 2 weeks compared to a lifetime when you are put back together again and you are once again an okay person. For me it is hard to visualize anyone not wanting to have it done.

What advice would you like to give other women considering breast reconstruction?

I think it is important for women to know that they can look good again. They need to hear positive comments, not all of the stories about people dying. They need to know that they have options. It would be nice if women could understand the positive way that you feel after you have had this operation. The pain is nothing compared to the good feelings you experience after it is over. Tell them not to be afraid, to be willing to investigate reconstruction. Check with different doctors and feel good about the doctor who is doing it.

IDA: IT'S NEVER TOO LATE

Ida is a small, gentle woman in her early sixties, who speaks with a soft, Southern drawl. She grew up at a time when women took a back seat to men and did not verbalize their own needs. Ida was quite beautiful when she was young, and she has always been proud of her good looks. When she learned that she might have breast cancer and treatment of her cancer would result in the loss of her breast, she felt she might as well be dead. "If it were malignant, I just didn't want to wake up." Her biopsy revealed a breast malignancy, and in 1968 Ida had a radical mastectomy of the right breast. "When I say radical, I mean radical. In 1968, they really took everything; they took most of the tissue under the arm and the nodes and they left you stripped and scarred. I was considered quite pretty at that time and I was a little vain, but after the surgery was over I was completely defeated. I really didn't care about living anymore. I thought, "Who could love anybody like this?"

Through the support of her husband and friends, Ida did eventually recover. She got a prosthesis and resumed her life. But negative feelings were still present. The scar tissue was a daily reminder as she bathed or undressed for the night. "I knew that I was scarred and kind of ugly and it deflated me." Thus, when she heard about the option of breast reconstruction at a Reach to Recovery meeting, she went ahead and scheduled an appointment with a plastic surgeon who had been recommended by a friend who had the surgery. By this time it was 1979, 11 years after her original surgery, and few people realized how much this deformity still bothered her. Impressed with the demeanor and skill of the plastic surgeon she visited, Ida decided to have her breasts reconstructed. In late 1979 she had her right breast reconstructed with a latissimus dorsi flap and a silicone implant was placed under the muscle. During the same operation, a prophylactic mastectomy was performed on her left breast, and an implant was placed under the pectoralis muscles for an immediate breast reconstruction.

Unlike the other women interviewed, Ida's reconstruction was not successful. Her breasts were not symmetrical, her scars were wide, and hard, fibrous capsules formed around the implants. Her skin pulled and her breasts became very uncomfortable. Unwilling to accept her discomfort, Ida spent the next few years talking to her plastic surgeon about what could be done to improve her breast appearance. By that time new procedures were available for reconstruction, and he explained the possibility of using her stomach fat to reconstruct her breasts, thereby eliminating the hard silicone implants that reacted unfavorably with her body. In November 1982, Ida once again had reconstructive breast surgery. This time both breasts were reconstructed with rectus abdominis flaps and Ida was thrilled with the results. "It was fantastic. I came out with a beautiful bikini scar on my stomach. He even took away an old scar that looked terrible. You should see my scar and the two lovely breasts with a lot of that ugly scar tissue removed. I am very happy with what he has done for me. I'm so glad that I didn't give up."

Ida's story is an unusual one; she had two types of reconstructive surgery. When the first was unsuccessful, she was willing to try again. Married at the time of her mastectomy and first reconstructive breast surgery, Ida is now divorced and works as a receptionist. She is not a wealthy woman, and even though she has been paying on a small, personal insurance policy for many years, she found her insurance inadequate to cover the cost of her latest reconstructive surgery. Nevertheless, she was motivated to have this surgery despite her age or the expense, and she persevered and worked out a plan for paying for her breast reconstruction. Following are some insights that Ida was willing to share with me.

Why did you decide to have reconstructive breast surgery?

When you put on a pretty nightgown and you only have one breast, you either wear a tight bra all of the time or you appear lopsided. It makes you feel less feminine, less lovable. That is not a good feeling. I got tired of that feeling and wanted something more for myself.

When I was in the Reach to Recovery program, I heard about the possibility of breast reconstruction. They showed movies on it and had people talk to us about it and other treatments. Then I met some women who had their breasts reconstructed and they were very excited about it. One woman told me about her plastic surgeon and how she just loved him. She urged me to go talk to him. After I heard about reconstruction, I said to myself, "Why not me? Why shouldn't I do this. I want to be whole again." That is why I had my breasts reconstructed.

I have had a few people say, "We know that you did this to your breasts because you are vain and this operation is a cosmetic thing, just meant to make you look good." Well, I want to say to that, "Yes, in a way you are right. I think all women want to look good. Do you know any woman who wants to look bad? I don't. I want to look as good as I can for as long as I can." I am a survivor and I am a caring person about other people, but I care for me and that makes me care for you. That's why it was so important to be able to do this for me.

Why did you choose your plastic surgeon and did he meet your needs?

I learned of my plastic surgeon through a friend. He had done some surgery on her, and she was very happy with him. During my first appointment, I was impressed by his seemingly real desire to help me. I had several other consultations with him and each time I felt even better about him. He is a caring man, very sensitive to both your physical and mental needs. When I had my mastectomy, I had two surgeons who were concerned and helpful and tried to be understanding, but they weren't successful. They were not attuned to my mental needs; they were only concerned with my physical health. I wanted a plastic surgeon who cared about both. I have been pleased with my choice.

He has an untold amount of perseverance and understanding with me. If I needed to have my head severed, and he was going to do it, I would go into the surgery with all of the confidence in the world. That is how much faith I have in him. His understanding was as important to me as his skill in surgery, because he had to understand me to give me the support I needed to get through surgery.

He demonstrated his support by always having time to explain anything that I wanted to know. He listens and answers my questions, no matter how minute or how detailed they are. I appreciate that; I know that this is a busy world we live in and I know that doctors are swamped. Everybody is head over heels in high gear, and it is wonderful to have someone who does not say, "Number please."

What went wrong with your first reconstructive surgery with the latissimus dorsi (back muscle) flap?

With my first reconstruction, I really had two different surgeries. The radical mastectomy deformity of my right breast was reconstructed with my latissimus dorsi back muscle and a silicone implant was inserted under the muscle. Then, a prophylactic mastectomy was performed on my left breast to guard again the development of future cancer in that breast, and my plastic surgeon inserted a silicone implant to reconstruct this breast. I was not happy with the results of my reconstructive surgery. The left breast pulled against the right. My scars healed well, but they were wide and I wasn't satisfied with the way they looked.

I had down days, and I had discomfort from my implants. They were hard and they were heavy and they made my skin feel tight and pulled. My breasts did not feel natural. Nothing I did to them made them feel any better. I tried massage and exercise, but they remained firm and hard. I also had all of this ugly scar tissue that had formed.

Have you had any complications with your second reconstruction with the lower abdominal flap and no implants?

I have had no problems at all. My breasts are soft and natural. There's nothing artificial; it's all me.

After complications developed with your first breast reconstruction, why did you go back to the same plastic surgeon for your second reconstruction?

Well, I wasn't happy with the way I looked, but I was happy with him. He had done a magnificent job. If he hadn't done a good job, I would have been all botched up, but I wasn't. The implants were heavy and hard and scar tissue formed, but he couldn't prevent my body's reaction to the implant. He has always tried to help me. There are, I'm sure, many wonderful doctors in the world, but there are very few doctors who have his special talent. He lets you know that he cares. I went back to him because I knew he would be honest with me and he would help me.

Was your reconstructive surgery painful and how long did it take you to recuperate?

I did not experience much pain with either of my reconstructions. The second one, with the rectus abdominis muscle, was actually easier than the first, but I sailed through both of them very well.

With my first reconstruction, when they used the back muscle, my daughter had more problems than her mother. She had never seen anyone who had been in surgery before and so when they brought me back into the room, she thought I was dying. They had to take her out and give her a tranquilizer. The next morning I was feeling better. In fact, I noticed that they had taken the nail polish off my toenails and fingernails and I said to my daughter, "Oh, Susan darling, get the nail polish and fix my nails." This was the next day, so you know that I couldn't have been in too much pain. I had drains in me and during this first reconstructive surgery my daughter stayed with me in the hospital for the 5 days I was in. She never left the hospital. With my second reconstructive surgery, using the stomach fat, she came and stayed overnight and the next day. Then she said, "Mother, you are doing so great. Is it all right if I go home?" I said sure, because I really didn't need anyone. I felt great. I was in the hospital for 9 days.

Are you satisfied with the physical appearance of your reconstructed breasts?

Yes, with this reconstruction I am. My scars are beautiful. I believe my plastic surgeon even has a portfolio of pictures of them; we're so proud of them. My breasts are soft and they match. I have a lovely bikini scar and some of the ugly scar tissue from my mastectomy has been removed. Also, my chest is filled in and I don't have that hollow look anymore.

How did your family react to your decision to have breast reconstruction?

My family never wanted me to do it. It wasn't that they didn't want me to get my breasts back, they were just afraid of my being put to sleep and the things that happen in hospitals.

How did you pay for your reconstructive surgery each time?

My first reconstruction was covered by insurance. I was working for the state at the time and had coverage through work and through an individual insurance policy that I had. Between the two policies, the total cost of hospitalization and surgery was paid for.

For my second reconstruction, I was no longer with the state, but my plastic surgeon worked with me. He said that he would only charge me for what my insurance would cover; it was a personal insurance policy that I had been paying on for many years. I did have a balance left on my hospital bill, which I myself am paying off in monthly payments.

Why after so much surgery did you decide to have your nipple-areola reconstructed?

I wanted to be a total person with nipples and everything, so I needed that nipple. I was amazed at how simple the procedure was. I let my doctor do it in the office. He went in there and put the nipple on, and I didn't even know when. He said, "Well, you are all finished now, and I want you to lie there 40 minutes and rest." I said, "Gee, I didn't even know that you had finished yet." Everything went fine, and I am very pleased with it.

Was your reconstruction worth all of the time, pain, and money? Would you do it again?

I am very happy with what I had done. Breast reconstruction makes you feel whole again. You don't feel ugly anymore. Every woman wants two breasts of her own. You came in with two and you want to go out with two. Even though I've been through a lot, I would definitely do it again.

Reconstruction had produced some changes in me. I dress more freely. I can wear anything I want to now. I was limited for so long. High-necked dresses, scarves, and long sleeves all constrict you.

I look good and it has made me feel good. My friends notice the difference. If I meet someone, and we become friends enough to talk about it, I tell them all about my reconstruction and they can't believe it. They will reach over and say, "Can I touch you?" They touch me and say, "I don't believe it; you feel just like me." and I say, "Yes, I am just like you. That's me. That's fatty tissue from my stomach, and it is all me. I don't have an implant." They marvel at it; so do I.

Some days I feel as if the cancer and mastectomy never happened. I feel so good about my reconstruction that I now realize that my mental state is just as necessary and important as my physical well being, because the mental affects the physical. I would never have been happy or satisfied if I hadn't had breast reconstruction. It has done wonders for me.

What advice would you like to give to other women considering breast reconstruction?

For all the ladies that have to have mastectomies, I would like to tell them not to ever feel that you cannot still be beautiful. You can have the breast restoration. It doesn't hurt too much and you will be proud of yourself for having had the courage to do it. Just do it for yourself, because it makes you feel wonderful after it's over. Don't wait all those years and suffer in silence. We don't have to do that anymore. Today, there is a new beginning, and women don't have to sit in the back seat and listen. They can speak up and be heard.

I grew up in a time when women were seen but not heard. But I think you have to stand up for what you want. I took responsibility for my own body. There are many women who would say, "Oh, I couldn't do that. My husband wouldn't approve." My question to you is, "Why does he have to approve?" It's your body not his body. They don't kill you when they put on a new breast; they make you whole again and it's truly a wonderful thing to behold.

MARY: MY FAITH HAS KEPT ME STRONG

Dressed in a light, ruffled summer dress, Mary was sitting in a chair in the doctor's office waiting for our interview. She was holding a copy of the New Testament in her lap and was busy working on a needlework picture. I noted how straight she sat as she waited, not realizing that she was trying to counteract the pulling she was feeling from her reconstructive breast surgery, performed only 6 weeks earlier. Tall, dark haired, and slim, Mary, a devout Baptist, spoke to me in a quiet determined voice as she related how her faith in the Lord had sustained her throughout her ordeal with cancer.

Five and one-half years ago, when Mary was involved with a busy life as a physical education teacher, coach, mother of two, and wife and "under a good deal of stress," she was diagnosed as having breast cancer. To treat her cancer, Mary had a modified radical mastectomy on her left breast, followed by 13 months of chemotherapy. She freely admitted that the chemotherapy was difficult to cope with because, as Mary said, I'm kind of a health nut. I'm usually on health programs and I believe in using vitamins. I know that chemotherapy is poison, and I didn't like it. But I accepted it because it was what the Lord had for me."

During her chemotherapy treatment, Mary heard about reconstructive surgery and wanted to learn more about it. She had read about this option in some popular magazines and went to see a plastic surgeon about it. She did not like the first doctor she consulted, and she also discovered that she could not have reconstructive surgery while she was still undergoing chemotherapy. But she decided that if the Lord wanted this for her, she would seek reconstructive breast surgery when she was ready for it. Then she would find a doctor and a procedure that met her needs. Five years later (the time that her general surgeon had suggested she wait) she had her breasts reconstructed. Because she had a flabby stomach that was of great concern to her, Mary chose the most complicated and extensive of reconstructive procedures to not only restore her breasts but to tighten her stomach at the same time. She had her left breast reconstructed with a rectus abdominis (stomach muscle) flap; a prophylactic mastectomy (to remove tissue in danger of becoming cancerous) and reconstruction were performed in her right breast with the right half of the lower abdominal flap. Today, at age 41, Mary is ready to schedule the next stage of her surgery to adjust her breasts for symmetry and reconstruct her nipple-areola. Mary's story, as she related it to me, is a particularly interesting one.

Why did you decide to have breast reconstruction?

I would think that anyone who has had a breast removed would want to consider breast reconstruction. You hear about it on TV; you read about it everywhere. It is more of a commonplace happening now and not a rarity. People know more what to expect. For me, I wanted breast reconstruction to feel whole again and to have my breasts back. Knowing that there was a reconstructive procedure that would also allow me to have a flat stomach provided a double reward; that is probably what prompted me more than anything else to take the plunge and say, "I'm going to do it."

After my mastectomy, I hated taking showers, and I hated getting out of the shower in front of the big mirror (which is almost always there in bathrooms). I definitely hated being naked at any time. I wasn't comfortable being naked in front of my husband, even though he accepted me beautifully and had nothing but encouragement for me. I still didn't like it; there was an ugly scar there. I was deformed looking. I tried not to think about it any more than I had to.

In the summer, I thought about my deformity more when I went swimming and wore a bathing suit. You also have to have pouches put in your bras to hold your prosthesis. This may sound horrible, but I only had four bras in 5 years, because I would just wear them and wear them until they would fall apart before I would make the effort to go buy any more and get another pocket sewn in and go through all of that. I disliked having the prosthesis in the summer, because it was hot, and if I did anything active, my prosthesis would cause a heat rash. When I would work in the yard and lean over to pull weeds, the prosthesis would be hot and heavy and it would hang on me. If I looked down, I could see all the way to my belly button. So, I couldn't, except in my yard, wear anything that had any type of plunging neckline for fear that when I would bend over, my prosthesis would show.

I made my final decision to have breast reconstruction after much soul searching and prayer. I had prayed to the Lord all along that "If You would have me have reconstructive surgery, I want to do it." I knew it was not a small decision to make, and I do not want to do anything in my life if the Lord doesn't want me to do it. So I just laid it before him and said, "If this is what You think I should do, I want to do it."

How did you choose the plastic surgeon to reconstruct your breasts?

When I decided that I wanted to have my breast reconstructed, I got the name of a plastic surgeon from my internist and cancer doctor. Then, my husband and I set up an appointment to see him. We both went, but we didn't like his bedside manner; he was really out of it. He came bopping into the examining room, thinking I was going to have a breast augmentation. Obviously, he didn't take time to read my chart. He was bragging about how wonderful it was going to be and what he was going to do for me. I just looked at him and thought that this doesn't make sense. I said, "I'm here to talk about breast reconstruction." Then his face turned white, and he apologized about the way he entered the room and about his attitude. After that he went into his reconstruction routine and explained that in order to create a new breast he would need to use my back muscle (latissimus dorsi) and he would bring it around to my front. He said he would request my hospital records, and we should come back for another consultation.

We came back a second time; but I was still not happy with him. He talked to me privately without my husband. He seemed to think that it was my husband's idea that I have the reconstruction and not mine, and he was concerned about that. Then he talked to my husband privately and he just aggravated both of us. Something as important as that wouldn't be anything a husband would drag a wife into a doctor's office for and say, "We want this done." When the consultation was almost over, he told me I couldn't have reconstruction right then anyway, because I was still undergoing chemotherapy. But it took two visits before that information came out. I wasn't in the mood to fool with him after our two conferences because I just didn't like him that much and I couldn't have it done anyway. So I just put it aside and decided to wait.

One year ago, I ran into a friend who had a mastectomy 3 years before me, and she said, "I'm so excited because I'm going to have my breast reconstructed." She told me about her doctor, and I said, "Great! I want to talk to you afterward and you can tell me how you like your surgeon." Some time later I saw her at the grocery store, this was after she had her surgery, and she said it was wonderful and she was so much happier. I took her doctor's name from her. Then I called my cancer doctor and got two more names. I sat with the three names trying to figure what to do, and I decided to call the one who I knew the most about. So I called his office and made an appointment.

When I met him, I liked him immediately. He has a gentle, patient, loving personality. He listens to you. He smiles at you. I chose him because he was recommended, he had ability, and he had a good bedside manner that revealed real love and concern. You want to be able to feel that your doctor really cares about you and that you can talk to him.

Most doctors are brilliant. Unfortunately, most brilliant people do not have a human side of love and compassion for people because these qualities don't seem to come in the same combination. So when you do find compassion and talent in a surgeon, you really want to latch on to him and enjoy your association because he is a rare find. It is definitely a blessing from the Lord to combine the two.

How could your plastic surgeon have helped you more?

He was wonderful and caring, but he probably could have communicated better with me. When I told him that he didn't tell me that the operation was going to be so hard, he said, "I told you it was going to be 'big surgery,' " and he did. I guess anyone knowing that she was going to have 4 hours of surgery would know that a lot would be involved, but I really didn't know what "big" entailed. I didn't know anything. He has done hundreds of operations. I would have liked to have had a little more information. I said once or twice during my recuperation that I wish my doctor could experience this pain so he could know what I am going through, and then maybe he would have prepared me a little better. But he's a man, and he doesn't think of the things women do and of the things that they wish they had been told.

Why did you choose to be reconstructed with the most complicated and extensive procedure you could select? Why didn't you select a simpler procedure that involved less time for recuperation?

I have always had a stomach, especially since my second child because I had a cesarean section, and it left me with a scar and a bowl of flab on my stomach. I hated my stomach and felt it was really ugly. My husband never liked it either; he never really criticized it, but I just knew that he didn't like it. His feelings made me dislike it even more. I really didn't like being in the nude.

To me it seemed huge; other people didn't even notice that I had it. They didn't see me when I was nude and all the flab was hanging out. I had even jested with my mother about having my stomach moved up to my breast, not having any idea that this could really be done.

When I was in the doctor's office and he was checking me, he told me to pull my panties down, because he wanted to see my stomach. Then he felt all that nice flab and he said, "This is what I would like to do," and he went into his language filled with medical terms and told me about moving the stomach muscles up and using the flab to make a new breast. I was so ecstatic that he could do a tummy tuck on me as well as give me a new breast that I could hardly contain myself.

I left the doctor's office and I was absolutely flying high. I was so jubilant that I thought, "Lord, I cannot believe it. You promised to work things out in life for our good. You promised to take the good and the bad things and use them to strengthen us and to make our lives better, but I cannot actually believe this. You are going to take this stomach away that I despised so desperately and move it up and give me a breast." I was just praising the Lord. My plastic surgeon had told me that it was the biggest operation I could have and would take about 4 hours to perform, but that didn't discourage me. It was just what I wanted. As I left his office I thought to myself, I bet he thinks I am an absolute kook. Here is a woman who has come in for breast reconstruction, and she is more excited about getting a flat stomach than she really is about getting her breast back.

Why did you decide to have a prophylactic mastectomy to remove the tissue from the normal breast before any diagnosis of cancer?

That was a difficult decision. I had to decide what to do with my good breast: whether to leave it alone or whether to let him go in, clean it out, and redo it. He could move the muscle up and repack this breast with stomach muscle and tissue. This muscle and tissue would only be available at the time of this surgery; it would never be available again. Because I had had one breast cancer, the chances for developing another tumor in my normal breast were increased.

I asked my husband for his advice. I know the Lord leads me through my husband, and he helps me in every decision I make. My husband said we should follow the doctor's recommendation. The doctor felt that since the tissue would be available, and because this would also be the wisest thing to do in the long run, that he would recommend the prophylactic mastectomy. So, on faith, I said, "Okay, this is what I'll do."

I questioned myself a couple of times after surgery and asked, "Did I do the right thing?" I could have had a breast with feeling there; now it's completely numb. It has a beautiful shape, however, and I am real pleased with everything they did to it. I just trust that what I did was the right thing for me.

Was your reconstructive surgery painful and how long did it take you to recuperate?

When I had my mastectomy, my pain was located in my arm. I really didn't want to move my arm at all. The pain with my reconstruction was from my breasts down to my pubic area. I don't know if there was a difference in intensity, but the reconstruction was worse because there was so much involved and any movement was hard. With my mastectomy, I could at least get up and move. My pain with my reconstruction was helped knowing mentally that I had a good reconstruction and that it was positive surgery which was going to make me more beautiful.

Twenty-four hours after my reconstructive surgery, when the catheter was still in me, the pain was pretty bad, but the pain shots helped. Once the catheter was out, I had a hard time going to the bathroom; it took another 24 hours before I could go normally. Two or three days later, with the help of the pain shots, I felt much better and my spirits were up.

In the meantime, they were getting me up to walk. Everything hurt. I couldn't stand up straight. I was stooped over worse than a 100-year-old woman and walking was hard.

After I came home from the hospital, I had one more pain pill, and then I never took anything else for pain. I decided that I could live without it. I don't like taking medicine, and I knew that if my head were clear I would feel better mentally.

My recuperation was hard because so much was involved. I couldn't move. I couldn't sleep except on my back. I had to work with my knees to get comfortable and had to pull the pillows under me. All I could do was just lay there. Getting up was awful. During the first three nights home from the hospital, I slept in my recliner and I was not comfortable. Sneezing and coughing just about killed me. It took about 2 weeks before I was sleeping normally again.

Fortunately, I have a Lazy Boy Recliner at home and when I got home I found my place on that chair and there I would sit. By then I could get comfortable if I could get in a certain position that was mostly sitting, with no strain or pressure on my body. I would get up to go to the kitchen or to the bathroom. I couldn't even carry a glass of water in my hand because that much weight just made me ache. I didn't realize the pain that I was going to have from the muscles that he flip flopped up. I was pretty helpless. I lived in and out of that chair for the second week.

At that time I developed some fluid buildup in my abdomen and when I consulted with the doctor he told me I should be as active as possible. So on the twelfth day after surgery I went with my family to an indoor farmer's market, and I got out and walked up and down the aisles. I walked slowly and bent over and I thought, "So what, I've got to start somewhere." I'm sure people looked at me and thought, "What's wrong with that woman?" Even so, I looked good; I had my makeup on and my hair looked nice. I felt as if I looked as nice as I could look even if I were stooped over. My spirits were ecstatic; getting out was the best thing that I could have done. I continued to be active and 2 weeks after surgery I was told that I could drive. At 4 weeks I started walking 30 minutes a day. I could have started earlier, but the weather was bad and I couldn't tolerate the cold, because it made my incisions hurt worse. Once I started walking, everything went faster. I could straighten up and each week I got a little straighter. I have probably been straight now for 3 weeks. Six weeks have passed since my surgery, and I feel fully recuperated.

Did you have any complications as a result of your surgery?

Twelve days after surgery I noticed that my stomach was a little wavy, and I thought, "They took the drains out but the fluid is still in me." I didn't like it because I knew it wasn't supposed to be there. Nobody told me to expect that fluid might build up. So I called the hospital and talked to the P.A. (physician's assistant) and told him that I had fluid in my abdomen and it was jiggling around. He told me that I wasn't active enough. So, I spent the day moving around, but when I looked at my abdomen that evening it was even more bloated. This caused me a bit of alarm. My stomach looked like a waterbed. I could poke it on one side, and it would ripple all the way across to the other side.

I called and was told by the doctor on call to come in so he could see it. I was apprehensive and disappointed. I didn't want to have a needle stuck in my abdomen after all I had been through. Anyway, nothing hurt. I came in and he drained me just by mashing the fluid out. He put a new drain bottle in me which I brought home with me and wore for another week or two because I had that much more fluid still draining. My doctor explained that I was having so much drainage because the new skin that they had pulled down over the muscle was not adhering to the new muscle and fluid was building up between the two. Well that explanation helped me to understand what was going on, so the liquid didn't bother me as much. I had no pain involved, just a wobbly stomach. I had to see the doctor two or three times a week for the next 2 or 3 weeks to drain the liquid. He would insert a needle, but he found a place that was dead so it didn't hurt. He stuck the needle in and drew off the fluid. Gradually my fluid disappeared and at the end of the 6 weeks I didn't have any left. I asked him if most people have this drainage problem, and he said that only 10% to 30% of them do. I had no other problems or complications from my surgery.

Are you satisfied with the physical appearance of your reconstructed breasts?

Yes, I am, even though they will be better after this next surgery to make final adjustments and to add the nipple. My scars are not objectionable and they will fade as time passes. My breasts actually look better than they did before surgery.

Why have you decided to have your nipple-areola reconstructed?

I am not a person who can accept a job halfway through. If I am going to do anything, I will do it all the way and in the best way possible. I just wouldn't be complete without a nipple-areola. I've gone through the worst and so to do that now is nothing.

When I have my nipple work done, he is going to adjust my breasts so that they are more symmetrical. I may have a small silicone implant put in under the muscle in both breasts. Right now the reconstructed breast does not look like the one that had the prophylactic mastectomy, even though they are packed with the same amount of fat. After he reshapes my breasts, they will look a lot better. I am actually looking forward to this next surgery.

Has reconstruction affected your sex life?

Yes, it has. I think that most men are excited with a woman's new body after breast reconstruction. I found my husband to be more sexually inclined. If I told him this, he would deny it, but I think that my reconstruction has helped him and given him more desire to have sex. He has enjoyed the fact that I now have a new breast back that had not been there for a long time. I think that men should not expect sex too quickly after a woman has had reconstruction. Women need some time to recuperate. They still feel protective of their bodies. I know that I still protect my body and breasts during intercourse.

How did you pay for your reconstructive surgery and was it covered by insurance?

I was working when my cancer was discovered, so my insurance bought the prosthesis. We were under double insurance at the time, which was a blessing. His insurance policy said we will either pay for the prosthesis *or* reconstructive surgery, so we just put the reconstructive surgery away and said, "Okay, we've got it paid for in the future when I'm ready." All we had to pay was $500 and they are paying 100% of the rest for the surgery and the hospital bill. I know that the hospital bill was $5000, but I don't even know what my plastic surgeon's bill is. I need to ask him how much it costs. All I was concerned about was if it were covered.

Was reconstructive surgery worth the pain, time, and money?

I would do it again. I am so happy with what has been done. My husband laughs at me because every time I pass the mirror I look at myself and I stare at my flat stomach first. I am so pleased to have a flat stomach. Then I look at my breasts, and I know that my breasts are not finished yet. Actually, I have had as much enjoyment out of my flat stomach as anything, and it's probably gotten me through this hard time more than knowing I have a breast, or maybe it's the two combined.

For me this reconstructive technique has really meant a lot. Even though my surgery was the biggest that you could have, I wouldn't do it any other way. I wanted the tummy tuck; it has done wonders for my self-image. I guess most women don't like their stomachs and are willing to pay the price to get rid of them.

I have both of my breasts now and I am normal again. Not only am I normal, but I'm better than I was before I had my breast surgery. My stomach is flat and my breasts look nicer and are bigger than the breasts that I had before. My chances of developing a breast cancer in my normal breast have also been reduced. I am very, very pleased. It was harder than the mastectomy, but mentally it was positive and that made you able to bear the pain better. I would do it again. I would recommend it being done for any person who had a desire for it.

ROBERTA: I HID IT FROM EVERYONE

"When I got divorced, 15 years after my mastectomy, I felt that I would never get married again, because no one would want to marry somebody who looked like I did. Although no one else was even aware that I had a mastectomy, I knew and I wouldn't risk letting anyone get close enough to me to discover my secret and see how ugly I really looked."

With these words, Roberta, a soft-spoken and gentle woman in her mid-forties began her conversation with me. Summarizing some of the real dilemmas facing women with mastectomies, she explained that she hesitated to get involved with men for fear of rejection. "When you get to be 40, there aren't that many men available to begin with; then, with your surgery, you place another obstacle in the way of friendship. It's a very precarious situation."

Roberta was only 23 and married when her cancer was discovered during a breast biopsy and she had a radical mastectomy on her left breast. Memories of this terrible experience continue to overwhelm her, and even as we talked she began to cry and then apologized for her tears. Roberta freely admits that she still feels bitter that she was denied a role in making the decision to amputate her own breast. Today, she strongly believes that women need information to enable them to make their own decisions about their bodies. "I was only 23 years old, just a baby, really. If I had been 40 or 50, maybe it wouldn't have been so bad. But they just did what they wanted to me. My feelings didn't matter; it was horrible. Afterward I didn't like to wear clothes, look at lingerie, or even hear people talk about their bodies, because it reminded me how ugly I looked." These feelings caused Roberta to hide her surgery from almost everyone, her children included, for 18 years until she learned about the option of breast reconstruction and decided to have her breast rebuilt.

When she got divorced, after 15 years of marriage, Roberta, the mother of three children, faced many of the usual worries of the single parent for rearing her children, supporting the family, and making a life for herself. Because she had a mastectomy, however, she had another set of problems to solve in trying to meet new people and possibly form new and lasting relationships. Worries about concealing her deformity were with her through all of these encounters.

Two years ago, Roberta learned of breast reconstruction and "It was like a miracle." She could not believe "that they could really do something for her." She had her breast reconstructed with a latissimus dorsi (back muscle) flap; her hollow chest was filled in and her axillary fold was recreated. To achieve symmetry, her remaining breast was augmented with a silicone implant placed under the muscle. A year after her breast was reconstructed, Roberta remarried.

In great part, Roberta attributes her ability to form a new and lasting intimate relationship to her decision to have breast reconstruction. "I never felt complete or really happy until I had breast reconstruction and that was 18 years later. It has made me a happier person. I was married at the time of my mastectomy, then later I was divorced, and now, approximately one year after my breast reconstruction, I have remarried. I think there's a message in there somewhere, and it might give some women hope."

How did you react to having a mastectomy?

I guess the mastectomy was the worst thing that has ever happened to me. When I went into the hospital, the doctor assured me that my lump wasn't anything to worry about, but, since he was going to do a D and C anyway, because of irregular menstrual periods that I was having, he would biopsy my lump at the same time. They put me in the hospital, did the biopsy, and didn't let me go home. The next night, the doctor told me he was going to remove my breast. He didn't ask me; I didn't sign anything. My husband signed the release. Nobody asked my opinion. They didn't care what I wanted; they just wheeled me in and cut off my breast. I was so heavily sedated when they told me, that I probably wouldn't have cared if they had said they were also going to amputate both of my legs.

When it was over, I was defeated. I felt totally helpless and out of control. If I had learned about my cancer in the doctor's office, with all of the facts in front of me, there is no doubt that I would have been unhappy and upset about this diagnosis, but at least I would have had an opportunity to confront my fears and make my own decisions. Probably, I would still have had a mastectomy, but it would not have been a radical and it would have been my choice.

Not long after my mastectomy, I read that Shirley Temple Black needed a mastectomy. Her doctor recommended that she have a radical mastectomy, but she was an intelligent woman, and she chose a modified radical. She is still alive. A woman, just like anyone else, should select the kind of surgery she wants to have. Physicians should draw on their knowledge of medicine to provide each patient with a reasonable and understandable explanation of her options and then let her weigh them in her own mind. If you are willing to take the chance of dying, that's okay, because it is your body.

Afterward, I discovered that my tumor was actually very small; it was still confined to local tissue and had not spread. Yet my surgeon did a radical mastectomy. He did too much. He told my mother and my family that I would hate him, and I did. Years later, after I had some information, I found that doctor and told him exactly what I felt. There were several different surgical approaches that he could have used, and at my age he should have given me a choice. He might think twice now before he does that to a woman again. What he did was a very "male" thing. My sister and I used to laugh about it later and speculate that if he had something that important to be cut off his body, he might have gotten a few opinions on it before he had it done.

How can people be more sensitive to mastectomy patients?

After my mastectomy, I was bothered by the way people are always discussing their bodies. Unfortunately, if you are a woman, you are not judged by your brain and that has always been difficult for me to accept. The culture that we live in is so body oriented that if you look in the mirror and your body appears ugly, it devastates you.

Right after I had my surgery, they came out with topless bathing suits. Now, I would never even want to wear anything like that. Still, I said "Oh Lord, here I am living in this day and time with this mutilated body and all people care about is the physical." Sometimes, I'd go into a bathing suit department and see all of those bikinis and have the hardest time. I would stand there and think or wonder, "If I hadn't had this surgery, would I have been brave enough to wear one of those?" I know that I wouldn't, but that is one of the things that bothered me.

How did your husband and family react to your mastectomy?

At first, I think everyone thought I was going to die because there had not been any cancer in our family before. My husband was kind, but overly protective and I became like a child. He was always trying to take care of me.

Do you feel that your mastectomy led to your divorce?

My husband said that the mastectomy didn't matter. He treated me pretty well even though our marriage didn't last, but our breakup was not caused by my surgery. I was the one who decided on the divorce and left him. Mostly, it was because we married awfully young; our marriage was not a happy one. I always felt that I would make the best of it, but you get to a point when you realize that you want more out of life.

Maybe surgery contributed to some of our problems. I always looked at myself and thought, "I was not like this when we got married, and maybe that is why we do not get along." I sometimes felt that deep down inside him my mastectomy caused some resentment toward me. Who knows? Maybe it did affect some of his feelings; I'm not sure. He never gave me any indication of that. I do know that the mastectomy affected my actions with him. He never saw my scar, I was less comfortable with my body, never undressing in front of him, and concealing myself from him the same way I hid my surgery from most everyone. I'm sure it didn't help us any.

Who did you tell about your mastectomy?

I was not one of those women who tells everyone what is wrong with her or what misfortunes have befallen her. Probably, I should have talked to a psychologist, but I tried to hide my problem because I was ashamed and didn't want anybody to know. The idea of having people feel sorry for me or think I was a freak was more than I could bear.

My mother, father, and sister knew and, of course, my husband. They were all very supportive. After my divorce, my sister was always introducing me to people and helping me to stay active and involved. I also told two of my very close friends. My friends treated me as if I were perfectly normal, even though I always felt a little different. Once one of my friends started to discuss someone she knew who had died of cancer, and then she looked at me and said, "Oh, I'm sorry," but my other friend said, "Don't be sorry for Roberta. There isn't anything wrong with her." They were just great.

How did your surgery affect your children?

It never really affected them at all. My twins were babies when I had the surgery, and my daughter was born 3 years afterward. I didn't ever tell them, because I was afraid they might think I was going to die young. So I kept it from them until I decided to have the breast reconstruction, 18 years later. When I told them, they couldn't believe it. My daughter said that she thought at one time she saw one of my bras with a patch, but she wasn't sure. That was the only time she ever thought of it. I never let them see. So it didn't affect them directly at all; even though my efforts to hide it might have made me a more nervous person to be around.

After your divorce, were you interested in dating again?

After the divorce, I moved with my three kids to be close to my family and for the support that they could give me. My chief concern was making a home for my children and getting them educated. And I did it; my children are now in college. My life was not important at that time. I got a job as a financial manager in an insurance company, and I was able to provide for my family and keep my life together. I didn't care about having a social life. I had girlfriends, but the thought of a relationship with a man never entered my mind. In fact, I never expected to get married again. I never even thought I would date. I'm serious; that is the honest truth. I just felt ugly about my surgery, and if it hadn't been for my loving and outgoing sister fixing me up with different friends, I would never have gone out.

Once you started dating, what were the problems you faced in forming new relationships with men?

For the most part, I never let it go that far. I was careful not to have any involved relationships, so the men I dated did not know about my surgery. Dating had a positive effect on me. All of a sudden, it dawned on me that "Goodness, they think I'm attractive." And I would go dancing and out to dinner, and there was one man that I probably could have gotten involved with but I wouldn't let myself. I was naive, and I hadn't had a serious relationship with any man other than my first husband because we had been married so long. But these men I was dating felt I was attractive, and I thought, "Well, he is interested in me," and it made me feel good, so I looked at myself a little differently. But all of the time, I wondered what would happen if I would meet a man and I told him about my surgery? And then, it happened.

What was the man's relationship to you and his reaction to finding out about your mastectomy?

I was introduced to him by my sister. He was divorced after an unhappy marriage. We became good pals. We would go everywhere together and had many of the same interests. We dated for a long time before we became sexually involved. He was not a worldly man. It's hard to believe it, in this day and age, but he was almost as naive as I was about sex. I told him about my mastectomy, and he said that it didn't matter to him.

How did you tell him about your mastectomy?

It was very difficult to tell him. We were talking about beauty and religion. He was very religious. I said that I believe in God, but I can't be very religious because of some of the things that have happened to me in my life. I said, "I was always the child that never did anything that my mother told me not to do. I was a virgin when I got married and look what happened to me." Then I told him everything and he couldn't believe me.

My mastectomy didn't seem to matter to him. He accepted me and thought I was attractive. In fact, when he discovered that I was contemplating breast reconstruction, he said "Are you sure that you want to undergo all of that pain? I think you look just fine." Of course, he had never really seen me. I always kept some distance, and I never let him look at me without something covering me. I just couldn't have done that.

Did you have an intimate relationship? And if so, how did you manage that without letting him see you?

Yes, we were intimate, but I always had a nightgown on and the room was darkened. The worst part of having the surgery is that you just don't feel feminine. My friend didn't make me feel that way; those feelings were self-inflicted. The first time we made love I kept asking myself what I was doing there. I didn't want to expose myself and I was terribly self-conscious. He would say, "It doesn't matter to me," and I'd say, "but it matters to me." I always wore a short nightgown. I just couldn't do it without it.

Considering how I was brought up, it was amazing for me even to get involved with a man. I'd have these conversations with myself and I'd think, "What are you doing?" Then I'd answer, "You're not getting any younger." Considering all of these problems, I had a fairly good relationship with this man, but there was always a strain for me there, because I felt self-conscious.

Why did your relationship with this man end? Do you think it had anything to do with your mastectomy?

No, not really. I'm not sure why it ended. He just broke it off, and I was upset for awhile. Now, when I think about it, I wonder why I had a relationship with him in the first place. Our personalities were completely different. In retrospect, the reason I thought he was wonderful was probably because he accepted me and my body didn't seem to make any difference to him. But at the time, I was emotionally involved, and I overlooked all of the negative aspects of his personality. If it weren't for my mastectomy, I might never have been attracted to him. Friends would always tell me, "You don't belong together," and I would say, "You just don't understand. He treats me so wonderful." I guess I felt lucky that any man would want to be with me. It didn't matter if he were my type or not; I couldn't be picky anymore. That's awful, but that's the way I felt.

Why did you seek reconstruction?

Because I always felt horrible. I guess the mastectomy was the worst thing that ever happened to me.

When I started dating men, I decided that I had a life other than being a mother and raising my children. I could actually have a close relationship with a man again and maybe even get married. In order to do that, I wanted to look as normal as possible. I wanted to please a man and have as good a physical and emotional relationship as I could. I don't think you can develop intimacy with someone if you are always worrying about how you look or about how he will react when he sees your scarred chest.

Why did you wait so long to have your breasts reconstructed?

I didn't know that reconstruction was even possible for someone with a radical mastectomy. I went for almost 18 years with no hope. The years just passed and after I moved with my children, I learned of this operation from my aunt who saw my plastic surgeon on educational TV. She was all excited when she called me on the telephone. She kept on raving about how absolutely amazing this surgery was. It was like a miracle.

I couldn't believe that a plastic surgeon could actually do something for me, and I told her that I was sure this operation was only for women who have had simple mastectomies. But she said, "Oh, no, you should have seen it! They showed all different kinds." I said, "Jean, I'm sure that those women were not as bad as I look," and she said, "They had all kinds and all ages. They had elderly women and very young ones." Just hearing about the different ages was reassuring to me. I always worried about my age; I always felt that I was the youngest person who ever had a mastectomy. My aunt convinced me to make an appointment with this plastic surgeon.

It took me about 6 to 8 months to make arrangements. I needed to change insurance companies to get more favorable coverage for reconstructive surgery and to find the right doctor to do my operation. My sister and I investigated who would be the best doctor to do a breast reconstruction and everyone recommended this same plastic surgeon. My sister found out all about him and how successful he had been with this surgery. So by the time I went to see him, I was feeling very good about him and about the operation.

If you had it to do over again, would you have your breast reconstructed immediately after your mastectomy surgery, so you would not have to experience breast loss?

Yes, I wish I had known about reconstruction earlier. I would have gladly avoided the trauma of seeing myself without my breast. A friend of mine learned about the possibility of reconstruction before she had a mastectomy, and she was told that she could have her breast reconstructed at the same time as her cancer surgery or later if she wanted it. Her doctors actually gave her some choices. I guess that's what I wanted, some options. Knowing that 1 year after my mastectomy, I could have my breast reconstructed would have satisfied me. Instead, I felt hopeless. Nobody provided me with any encouragement. They would tell me, "You are so lucky that you are not dead." I didn't even know that reconstruction was possible until almost 18 years after my mastectomy. That's too long to wait.

**What type of reconstructive procedure did
you select?**

> I had a flap reconstruction. They took the latissimus dorsi back
> muscle and used it to build a breast mound and to fill out my hol-
> lowed chest.

**Was your reconstructive surgery painful and how long did it
take you to recuperate?**

> I had more pain with my reconstruction than I had with my mastec-
> tomy. I stayed home about 3 to 4 weeks after reconstruction and
> then went back to work for a half day. My back hurt the most. I
> probably did too much after I got home. I am not one who likes to
> convalesce, and I tried to get active again, perhaps too quickly.
> Anyway, the scar pulled and when I went back 6 months later for
> a second operation to get a nipple-areola, my plastic surgeon rede-
> fined the scar so it wouldn't draw as much. The front of my chest
> and the new breast area didn't hurt at all. I was tired during re-
> covery, but it was also a happy time, because I kept thinking about
> how great I was going to look.

**Why did you choose to have your nipple-areola
reconstructed?**

> I wanted my breast to look as normal as possible and I never even
> thought about not having a nipple. It wouldn't be complete without
> it.

Did you have any surgery on your remaining breast?

> I had it augmented at the same time as my reconstruction so my
> breasts would match. I am glad I did it. In fact, I think it is a great
> boost to my ego. Anyone who is flat chested should consider an aug-
> mentation when she is getting her breast reconstructed. It makes
> you feel better.

**Are you satisfied with the physical appearance of your
reconstructed breast?**

> I figured that anything that he could do for me would be an im-
> provement. I'm very satisfied. My breast shape and contour look
> great. I'm not completely happy with some of the skin under my
> arm, because it hangs down a little and I still have scars in that area.
> But that's minor, and I don't want any more surgery right now. Re-
> construction doesn't make you have a perfect body, but oh, it's so
> much better than it was.

How did you pay for your reconstruction and was it covered by insurance?

Insurance covered most of it. It did not pay for the augmentation of my remaining breast. My plastic surgeon wrote letters to the insurance company explaining why I needed an augmentation, but they didn't care. We both called them and explained that I didn't ask for this procedure, but it was recommended. I only had the augmentation because I was flat chested and that was the only way my two breasts could be made to match. But, the insurance company still wouldn't cover it. When they see plastic surgery, I don't care how horrible the surgery is, they automatically think that the operation is purely cosmetic and something that you didn't have to do. They did pay for all of my reconstruction except for the deductible part and they paid for the second procedure to create the nipple.

How do people react when they learn that your breasts were reconstructed?

They think it is wonderful. My brother-in-law kids me all the time. My internist, whom I have been going to for years, even asked me if he could look. I showed him and do you know what he said. "Why, you could almost be in *Playboy*!" I thought that was real cute; it makes you feel so good. My mom was thrilled for me. She lived through all those years of my unhappiness, and even though she hated for me to have another operation, she knew that it was worth it. My dad was all for it also. They helped me when I came home from the hospital; the whole family did.

Was it difficult for you to seek more surgery after your initial experience with mastectomy had been so devastating?

No, it was exciting for me. I looked forward to it. When I was getting ready to go to the hospital I was overjoyed and later, even though it hurt, the pain really didn't bother me.

What are the benefits of reconstruction?

Reconstruction has been wonderful for me. I feel much better about myself. It's as if I am more complete now. Surgery has helped me to reach a point where I can have a good relationship with a man. I have regained my self-confidence and am less inhibited about my body. I feel more attractive and like a normal person again.

It's also a relief not to bother with that horrible prosthesis anymore. I couldn't wait to discard it. In fact, my mother threw them all away when I was in the hospital. Then she went out and bought me some lacy Bali bras, the kind with elastic and little support.

Before I had reconstruction, I felt as if my whole life were spent trying to find something that I could wear to conceal my mastectomy. I was very self-conscious. I hated to go shopping for clothes; every time I went it was an ordeal. Reconstruction has totally changed my attitude. Now, I enjoy shopping; I like to browse at clothes. Before, I avoided T-shirts with V necks or anything that might be revealing. I couldn't wear bathing suits unless I got them in a special store and I hated that. Now I can wear a little silk blouse and leave the first button open. There are still some things that I can't wear. But, oh my goodness, when I got married, I got some lingerie that you wouldn't believe. I can wear it and I look good in it. I love wearing frilly, feminine things like that again.

Did reconstruction affect your attitude toward men and marriage?

Yes, it made me more relaxed and willing to consider the possibility that I might be able to get married again. I still had some difficulty in confiding in anyone about my mastectomy or my reconstruction. When I met my present husband, I had already had breast reconstruction and was healed. I thought that I looked great, but still I worried about his finding out. I was afraid that if he knew maybe he wouldn't want to get involved with me. When he proposed marriage, I kept putting him off and saying, "But you don't know everything about me." We had made love (without my gown) but he still didn't know. You can tell how good my plastic surgeon is because when the lights are dim, you really can't tell. Finally, I told him, and it didn't make any difference to him. In fact he couldn't believe that my breast had been reconstructed; he thinks that I have the most wonderful doctor in the world.

Having the reconstructive surgery made me feel complete. If I hadn't had my breast restored, my husband would have still loved me, but it would have made a difference to me. I can give more freely now, and I am a better wife.

What advice would you like to give to women considering reconstruction?

I think that any woman who has a mastectomy or is considering one should learn about reconstruction. It does such positive things for you. Get all the information, look into several opinions, and locate the best doctor to perform this surgery. Investigate it fully; then do it for yourself. For the single woman, this procedure can do wonders. It can free you. Best of all, it restores your self-confidence and allows you to contribute to a relationship without self-consciousness and constraint.

Breast Cancer and Reconstruction Resources

AMERICAN CANCER SOCIETY

The American Cancer Society, Inc., is a national organization fighting cancer through numerous research and educational programs. Fifty-eight chartered divisions and nearly 3000 local units offer patient service and rehabilitation programs for cancer patients and their families, including information and guidance, donated and loaned equipment, rehabilitation programs (Reach to Recovery), literature, films, and speakers.

REACH TO RECOVERY

This American Cancer Society rehabilitation program for women who have had breast surgery is designed to help them meet their physical, psychological, and cosmetic needs. No meetings are held. On written referral from a physician, a trained volunteer, who has had a mastectomy, makes a hospital visit a few days after surgery, bringing a temporary breast form and providing information about rehabilitation. Information on breast reconstruction is usually available through this program. For more information, contact your local American Cancer Society.

I CAN COPE

This information seminar is sponsored by the American Cancer Society through area hospitals and offers (free of charge) eight sessions for cancer patients and their families on living with various aspects of cancer. The local American Cancer Society can be contacted for times, dates, locations, and registration information.

NATIONAL CANCER INSTITUTE (NCI)

For *free* literature write:

Publications Order—Office of Cancer Communications
National Cancer Institute
Building 31, Room 10A18
Bethesda, MD 20205
800-638-6694, 8 AM to Midnight

This organization offers free information to the general public and to professionals about cancer detection, diagnosis, and treatments and NCI-supported clinical trials and research programs.

BREAST CANCER ADVISORY CENTER

Rose Kushner, Director
P.O. Box 224
Kensington, MD 20895
301-984-1020

This volunteer group provides information on all aspects of cancer diagnosis and treatment.

CANCER RESEARCH INSTITUTE

133 East 58th Street
New York, NY 10022
800-223-7874
212-722-8547

This independent organization is medically and scientifically directed to select and support the most significant advances in cancer immunology research. It is a good resource for medical and research questions.

ENCORE (YWCA)

ENCORE National Board
YWCA
600 Lexington Avenue
New York, NY 10022

This group provides information on exercise for postoperative breast cancer patients. It also includes a discussion group. A woman can write to the above address or call her local YWCA branch to see if there is a group in her community.

MAKE TODAY COUNT

National Headquarters
514 Tama Building
Box 303
Burlington, IA 52601

A national organization with membership open to all persons with life-threatening illnesses and to their families and other interested persons. Groups meet monthly to share experiences and help each other to appreciate each day of life as it is lived.

AMERICAN SOCIETY OF PLASTIC AND RECONSTRUCTIVE SURGEONS

233 North Michigan
Suite 1900
Chicago, IL 60601
312-856-1818

This organization provides information on breast reconstruction and will give potential patients the names of three board-certified plastic surgeons practicing in their community.

APPENDIX B

A BREAST CANCER PATIENT'S OPTIONS AND RIGHTS*

- To receive a simple and clear diagnosis of her condition.
- To receive all available diagnostic procedures and a complete workup prior to surgery.
- To have the consent form clearly explained to her before she signs it.
- To have the biopsy performed first (under local anesthesia), including the right to see the pathologist's report and have it explained to her. Surgery may be performed at a later date.
- To be aware that for certain patients the future option of reconstructive plastic surgery exists and to have the surgeon take that option into consideration.
- To receive consideration from the surgeon and other medical personnel for the physical and emotional trauma she is undergoing.
- To receive an explanation of any viable alternative treatments—including biopsy with radiation therapy as primary treatment, chemotherapy, mastectomy, etc.—risks, disadvantages, and advantages of each treatment.
- To receive a satisfying explanation as to why the surgeon has decided on a particular surgical procedure rather than a less mutilating one.
- To be referred to a therapist for physical or psychiatric therapy following surgery.
- To receive competent follow-up care after surgery and to know who is going to be responsible for that care.
- To be referred to a support group for information and assistance with her personal concerns.
- To be always treated as an adult.

*Prepared by Women for Women, a nonprofit West Coast organization interested in the topic of breast cancer.

THE BREAST CANCER INFORMED CONSENT SUMMARY

Currently, several states require physicians to inform their patients of alternative treatments for breast cancer. In California physicians must provide that information in printed form: a seven-page pamphlet written in simple, nonmedical language, describing the various options (advantages and disadvantages) for breast cancer treatment with surgery, radiation, and chemotherapy.

The following is an example of that form:

BREAST CANCER TREATMENT
SUMMARY OF ALTERNATIVE
EFFECTIVE METHODS:
RISKS, ADVANTAGES, DISADVANTAGES*

January 1983

This summary is required by SB 1893, *The Breast Cancer Informed Consent Law*, effective January 1, 1981.

INTRODUCTION

You have a treatable disease and are entitled to know about the various medically effective surgical, radiological, and chemotherapeutic treatment procedures available.

This brochure has been developed to assist you to understand what these various treatment procedures are, their advantages, disadvantages, and risks.

The treatment of cancer is quite complex. It must be individualized. The choice of therapy may be difficult to make. It is important for you to have this basic information about the methods of treatment so that you may discuss them more fully with your physician as they apply to your case. This will help you understand what treatment programs may be used and what their effects may be in your individual situation. Using this information as a basis for discussion, you and your physician should be able to make an informed choice.

Because cancer is a serious disease, it may be appropriate for either you or your physician to seek additional opinions if either of you desires. Your consent is required before any treatment is carried out, and you have the right to participate in making the final choice of the treatment procedure(s). Your physician has a corresponding right to withdraw from the case if he chooses.

It is very important to take a reasonable amount of time to obtain enough medical information and consultation to make a final and informed decision. But prolonged delay may interfere with the success of your treatment. Making this choice is an important step. Once you and your physician have reached a decision about your treatment, you will have a positive attitude which will be a tremendous help as you and your physician begin and carry out the treatment of your cancer.

MANAGEMENT OF BREAST CANCER

Management of breast cancer is achieved by the cooperation of appropriate specialists in the field: the primary (personal) physician for general support and coordination, the surgeon for diagnosis by biopsy and specific surgical procedure for removal of the breast tumor, the pathologist for gross and microscopic diagnosis, the radiation oncologist for supervising and administering radiation treatment, and the medical oncologist for specialized management of the patient's care and administration of chemotherapy. In actual practice these members proceed fairly independently but maintain liaison by telephone and written reporting.

TREATMENT ALTERNATIVES: ADVANTAGES, DISADVANTAGES, RISKS

If your diagnosis is breast cancer, it is important for you to understand there is enough time to make a careful decision. Prolonged delay and failure to get adequate treatment may result in the deterioration of your situation. In contrast, the benefits of modern breast cancer therapy far outweigh the risks. This is especially true when treatment is undertaken early. The risk may be small or serious, and its occurrence may vary from frequent to rare. There is a wide range of potential benefits and risks from the various treatment procedures for the different stages and kinds of breast cancer. Before deciding on your course of therapy, you should discuss with your physician the particular benefits and risks of the treatment methods suitable for your individual case.

DIAGNOSIS

Diagnosis is the scientific determination of the nature of the lump. It is made by the pathologist who examines the tissue from the breast lump (breast biopsy) under the microscope.

The breast biopsy entails the surgical removal of part or all of the lump under suitable anesthesia. Unless the lump is quite large it is usually removed in one piece (excisional biopsy). (A large lump may be biopsied with a special needle or by surgically removing a small sample.) The tissue removed by biopsy provides material for the definitive test for cancer, namely, the examination of tissue under the microscope by the pathologist. If cancerous, part of the fresh tissue may also be studied for receptors for hormones (estrogen and progesterone), which could be important if future treatment decisions become necessary. (Only about 20% of breast biopsies are cancerous; the remainder represent less serious conditions.)

The procedure for obtaining the biopsy should be discussed with you, since you must make a decision between two courses of action—the one-step or two-step procedure.

In the one-step procedure, you and your physician decide beforehand that if the biopsy shows cancer and if surgery will be the treatment of choice, the entire procedure (biopsy, diagnosis by pathologist, and the appropriate surgery) will be completed in one operation.

In the two-step procedure, the biopsy is done under local or general anesthesia, and no additional operation is performed at this time. After the pathologist examines and reports on the biopsy, the surgeon reviews the pathology report with you and discusses with you the various treatment options available and effective for your particular case. A decision is then made by you and your physician on which procedure is preferred by you for your individual care.

Prior to the procedure you choose, a general medical evaluation which may include any or all of the following diagnostic procedures is usually done to determine your individual situation:

Your medical history (including family history of cancer)

Physical examination

Blood tests evaluating function of various systems, e.g., liver, kidney, immunity, etc.

X-ray films (chest, bones, etc.)

Breast x-ray films (mammography)

Radioisotope scan (bones, liver, brain, etc.)

Computerized tomographic body scans (specialized x-ray views of any or all internal organs and bones)

Sonograms (pictures of internal organs made with ultrasound waves)

Treatment recommendations are individualized. They are based primarily on the extent (stage) and type of disease present, as well as other factors related to your personal health.

SURGERY

This process involves removal of the tumor, and either a portion of the breast, all of the breast, or all of the breast and some surrounding tissues as well.

Radical (Halsted) Mastectomy

The radical (Halsted) mastectomy is not commonly used today except in unusual cases. In this procedure, the entire breast, nipple, some of the overlying skin, underlying chest muscles, nearby soft tissue, and lymph nodes extending into the armpit are removed.

Advantages. If cancer has not spread beyond breast or nearby tissue, it can be completely removed. Examination of lymph nodes provides information that is essential in planning future treatment.

Disadvantages. Removes entire breast and underlying chest muscles. Leaves a long scar and a hollow area where the muscles were removed. May result in swelling of the arm, some loss of muscle power in the arm, restricted shoulder motion, and some numbness and discomfort. Reconstructive (plastic) surgery and fitting of breast prosthesis are difficult.

Modified Radical Mastectomy

The entire breast, nipple, some of the overlying skin, nearby soft tissue, and lymph nodes in the armpit are removed. Chest muscles are left intact, but overlying covering of muscle is removed.

Advantages. Retains the chest muscles and muscle strength of arm. Swelling of arm occurs less frequently and is milder than after radical. Cosmetic appearance is better than with radical. Apparently as effective as radical, but not if cancer is large or has invaded the muscle sheath. Cosmetically effective reconstructive surgery is usually feasible.

Disadvantages. Entire breast and part of overlying skin are removed. In some cases removal of lymph nodes in armpit may be incomplete. Some persons may experience swelling of the arm.

Simple Mastectomy

The main breast structure, but not overlying skin, is removed. Underlying chest muscles and often armpit lymph nodes are left in place. Many surgeons remove some of the armpit lymph nodes through a separate small incision under the arm to determine if cancer has spread to nodes. Often followed by radiation therapy.

Advantages. Chest muscles are not removed and strength of arm is not affected. Swelling of arm occurs infrequently. Reconstructive surgery usually feasible.

Disadvantages. Breast is not preserved. If cancer has spread to armpit lymph nodes, it may remain undiscovered unless these nodes are sampled or removed at the time of surgery; adequate treatment could be delayed.

Segmental Mastectomy, Partial Mastectomy, and Lumpectomy

If cancer is small and detected early, a segment of the breast containing the tumor is removed. Many surgeons also remove some armpit lymph nodes through a separate incision to check for possible spread of cancer. Most cancer experts feel this type of operation should be followed by radiation therapy and some feel chemotherapy should be used in selected cases as well. These procedures are relatively new and long-term results are being documented.

Advantages. Most of the breast remains. Reconstructive surgery is usually easier if needed at all. Loss of muscle strength and swelling of the arm are unlikely to occur. Commonly used as first step for radiation therapy as primary treatment in early breast cancer, especially if preservation of the breast is desired.

Disadvantages. Most cancer specialists feel these procedures may be incomplete unless armpit lymph nodes are removed for pathological examination and person is given radiation therapy or a combination of radiation therapy and chemotherapy. Otherwise, spread of cancer into armpit lymph nodes or undetected areas of cancer present elsewhere in breast may go untreated and chance for cure may be lost.

RADIATION (X-RAY) THERAPY

Radiation treatment of local tissues of the body, known as radiotherapy, can destroy cancer cells while producing less injury to surrounding tissues. Radiation for treatment may come from a number of devices, e.g., super voltage x-ray, linear accelerator, Betatron, Cobalt-60 and radioactive isotopes. The source and type of radiation is chosen to suit the requirements of the individual.

Radiation Therapy as Primary Treatment in Early Breast Cancer

This approach has been used for about 10 years in this country and for about 20 years in Europe for the treatment of early breast cancer. After pathologic diagnosis by biopsy and surgical removal of the local tumor, external radiation therapy is used to treat the remainder of the breast, the lymph nodes, and the chest wall. This is then followed by a radiation "boost" to the biopsy site with radioactive sources temporarily introduced into the area of the excision. Sometimes the boost may be given with more external irradiation (or electron beam).

Advantages. The breast is preserved. It may be mildly to moderately firmer. Usually there is minimal or no visible deformity of surrounding tissues. After completion of the treatment, the skin usually regains normal appearance.

In early breast cancer, lumpectomy or segmental resection, with radiation as the primary treatment, has demonstrated results that currently appear equal to long established surgical procedures.

Disadvantages. A full course of treatment requires daily outpatient visits for 4 to 6 weeks. Treatment may produce a skin reaction similar to sunburn and may cause temporary difficulty in swallowing. Radiation therapy can affect bone marrow where blood cells are made. This may limit the dosage and effectiveness of later chemotherapy if it is needed. A small area of scarring, permanently visible on x-ray examination, may develop in the lung, but usually causes no symptoms.

Radiation Therapy as a Supplement (Adjuvant) to Surgery

Following surgery, examination of the surgical specimen by the pathologist may show the cancer has spread outside the breast and into armpit lymph nodes or local surrounding areas. Radiation therapy will usually control cancer cells remaining in these areas. The treatment of advanced cancer often requires the consultation and coordinated efforts of the surgeon, radiation oncologist, and medical oncologist.

Advantages. The goal of radiation therapy is to destroy cancer cells in tissue in the radiation treatment area which improves control of or stops the spread of cancer in the treatment area. Modern equipment gives very precise control of the x-ray treatment. Radiation therapy may be used to treat localized metastases.

Disadvantages. The major side effects are the same as those listed under radiation therapy as a primary treatment. When cancer is treated by radiation therapy as a supplement to surgery, there may be wide variations in the extent of the treatments required, depending on the problem or site of disease being treated.

CHEMOTHERAPY

The medical oncologist is the specialist who usually plans and administers the chemotherapy and may coordinate the patient's management with other physicians. Chemotherapy is designed to destroy breast cancer cells that cannot be removed surgically or by radiation or their combination.

In recent years important and effective advances in breast cancer treatment have been made in this area, especially advanced cancer. Different drugs or a combination of drugs are administered orally or by injection. This program is adapted to the individual and may continue at intervals for 6 months to 2 years or longer, depending on the cancer being treated and the drug program being used.

Supplemental (Adjuvant) Chemotherapy

Chemotherapy supplements primary surgical or radiation treatment when it is likely the patient has a cancer which has spread into or beyond nearby lymph nodes. Such patients have a higher risk of recurrence than those whose lymph nodes are found to be free of cancer.

Supplemental chemotherapy may reduce this risk considerably.

Advantages. Increases the effectiveness of surgery or radiation therapy and reduces the risk of breast cancer recurrence. Works to stop its growth at distant sites in the body.

Disadvantages. Most chemotherapy drugs have reversible side effects. Some side effects are minimal, while others can cause discomfort, including nausea, temporary loss of hair, bone marrow depression (resulting in temporary susceptibility to infection and bleeding tendency), anemia, loss of appetite, fatigue, and, rarely, damage to heart muscles. Also may depress reproductive function and cause change of life symptoms. Newer techniques of administration and dosage reduce the side effects of chemotherapy.

Chemotherapy for Recurrent Breast Cancer

Anticancer drugs, taken alone or in combination with other modalities, can arrest the disease, help to relieve symptoms, and prolong the life of a patient who experiences recurrence of breast cancer.

Hormonal Therapy

Many breast cancers are sensitive to female hormones (estrogen and progesterone) and are partially controlled by them. In many treatment centers, fresh tissue from the tumor (specimen or biopsy) can be tested to measure this hormone sensitivity (estrogen receptor assay). In some breast cancer patients, beneficial effects can be received by adding hormones, removing glands that produce them, or administering drugs (antihormones) that counteract the hormones produced by the body. Hormone therapy often increases significantly the effectiveness of other cancer therapy.

INVESTIGATIVE TREATMENTS FOR BREAST CANCER

Clinical trials are new treatments which are not yet generally available. Laboratory or other reliable studies may indicate a new cancer treatment procedure or therapy program could be better than ones in current use. Research to measure effectiveness is conducted in clinical trials by many major cancer treatment groups. The new treatment methods are put to general use only after long-term evaluation by cancer experts when they find the new treatment gives results as good as, or better than, established treatments.

BREAST FORMS

Breast forms (prostheses) are made with a variety of substances such as silicone, foam rubber, Silastic, viscous fluid, or glycerin. Fitted individually and worn in brassiere pockets, they can give the form, weight, and appearance of a normal bustline. The right bra for you may very well be the one you've always worn. Your health insurance generally covers a portion of this cost with your physician's prescription.

RECONSTRUCTIVE BREAST PROCEDURES

Reconstructive plastic surgery may effectively restore the form of the breast and adjacent tissues lost at surgery. Implants of breast prostheses or surgical transfer of body tissues may be used. Usually at least two surgeries are required to achieve desired results, but in some cases advance planning can minimize this. The possibility of reconstructive surgery should be discussed with your physician in advance of a definitive surgical treatment procedure. You should investigate the extent of financial coverage available through your health insurance for this procedure.

FOLLOW-UP

The success of cancer treatment depends not only on early detection and effective treatment, but also on a careful, consistent follow-up program to detect cancer recurrence as early as possible if it should occur. Consistent regular visits to the treating physician and monthly self-examination are essential. New methods of detection and treatment are being continually developed and can be used to your advantage.

Many very helpful and thoughtful women who have been through a similar experience can lend you their support and guidance. They can be contacted through your physician, your hospital, your local unit of the American Cancer Society, or the National Cancer Institute's Cancer Information Service.

SUMMARY

This brochure is intended to make you aware of the effective alternative methods of treating breast cancer available in California, and your role in choosing the method to be used in your care. In order to reach a decision on the treatment method, it is important for you to understand the nature of the disease, the extent of your problem, the treatment needed, the method or methods of providing that treatment suitable to your particular situation, and finally the results that may reasonably be expected.

This is best done by having a complete evaluation followed by a thorough discussion with your physician(s). The brochure should assist you to participate in these discussions by providing essential background information so you can ask questions you need answered, and help you understand what your physician is talking about and how the choice of cancer treatment method will affect you and your circumstances.

Many important details are necessarily left out, and you should look to your physician for your complete and current information. Being well informed and having thoroughly discussed the alternatives will make it easier to make a knowledgeable decision about your course of treatment. It will give you justified confidence you have made the best choice possible. This will be a tremendous help to you and your physician as you carry out your treatment and establish your follow-up program.

*Prepared by the State Department of Health Services based on recommendations of the State Cancer Advisory Council. Printed and distributed by the Board of Medical Quality Assurance, California Department of Consumer Affairs.

CLASSIFICATION SYSTEM OF BREAST CARCINOMA *

The following classification system, prepared by the American Joint Committee for Cancer Staging and End Results Reporting, describes the tumor, the condition of the lymph nodes, and the presence of metastasis individually and then combines that information to classify breast cancer into four stages. Under the AJC system, tumors (T) and nodes (N) are described both presurgically and postsurgically, because after pathological study their condition may change.

CLINICAL CLASSIFICATION OF PRIMARY TUMOR (PRESURGERY)

TX   Tumor cannot be assessed.

TO   No evidence of primary tumor.

TIS   Paget's disease of the nipple with no demonstrable tumor. (Paget's disease with a demonstrable tumor is classified according to size of the tumor.)

T1†   Tumor 2 cm or less in greatest dimension.
T1a: No fixation to underlying pectoral fascia or muscle.
T1b: Fixation to underlying pectoral fascia and/or muscle.

T2†   Tumor more than 2 cm, but not more than 5 cm, in its greatest dimension.
T2a: No fixation to underlying pectoral fascia and/or muscle.
T2b: Fixation to underlying pectoral fascia and/or muscle.

T3†   Tumor more than 5 cm in its greatest dimension.
T3a: No fixation to underlying pectoral fascia and/or muscle.
T3b: Fixation to underlying pectoral fascia and/or muscle.

---

*From The breast cancer digest: A guide to medical care, emotional support, and educational programs, Pub. No. 82-6191, Baltimore, 1982, National Cancer Institute.
†Dimpling of the skin, nipple retraction, or any other skin changes except those in T4b may occur in T1, T2, or T3 without the classification.

T4 Tumor of any size with direct extension to chest wall or skin. (Chest wall includes ribs, intercostal muscles, and serratus anterior muscle, but not pectoral muscle.)

T4a: Fixation to chest wall.

T4b: Edema, including peau d'orange (orange peel skin), ulceration of the skin of the breast, or satellite skin nodules confined to the same breast.

T4c: Both of the above.

T4d: Inflammatory carcinoma.

PATHOLOGICAL CLASSIFICATION OF PRIMARY TUMOR (POSTSURGERY)

TIS Preinvasive carcinoma (carcinoma in situ, noninfiltrating intraductal carcinoma, or Paget's disease of nipple).

Postsurgical TX, TO, T1a and b, T2a and b, T3a and b, T4a, b, c, and d are the same as clinical classification (presurgery).

CLINICAL CLASSIFICATION OF LYMPH NODES (PRESURGERY)

The following information is used to describe the condition of the regional lymph nodes (N):

NX Regional lymph nodes cannot be assessed clinically.

NO No palpable homolateral axillary nodes.

N1 Movable homolateral axillary nodes.

N1a: Nodes not considered to contain growth.

N1b: Nodes considered to contain growth.

N2 Homolateral axillary nodes considered to contain growth and fixed to one another or to other structures.

N3 Homolateral supraclavicular or infraclavicular nodes considered to contain growth or edema of the arm.

PATHOLOGICAL CLASSIFICATION OF LYMPH NODES (POSTSURGERY)

NX Regional lymph nodes cannot be assessed clinically.

NO No metastatic homolateral axillary nodes.

N1 Movable homolateral axillary metastatic nodes not fixed to one another or other structures.

N1b: Lymph nodes with only histological metastatic growth.

N1a: Gross metastatic carcinoma in lymph nodes.

N1bi: Micrometastasis smaller than 0.2 cm.

N1bii: Metastasis (larger than 0.2 cm) to one to three lymph nodes.

N1biii: Metastasis to four or more lymph nodes.

N1biv: Extension of metastasis beyond node capsule.

N1bv: Any positive node greater than 2 cm in diameter.

N2 Homolateral axillary nodes containing metastatic tumor and fixed to one another or to other structures.

N3 Same as for clinical classification.

CLASSIFICATION OF METASTASIS

Metastasis (M) is classified:

MX Metastasis not assessed.

MO No (known) distant metastasis.

M1 Distant metastasis present, specify site.

When all the information about the tumor, nodes, and metastasis has been assessed and combined, that information will provide the physician with the stage of disease. Disease stages are described as:

Stage I. A tumor less than 5 cm with minor skin involvement, either affixed or not affixed to the chest wall, muscle, or fascia; nodes not considered to contain growth; no evidence of metastasis.

Classified:	Tla	No, Nla	MO
	Tlb	No, Nla	MO

Stage II. A tumor less than 5 cm with possible muscle or chest wall fixation; nodes are movable, but may or may not contain growth; no evidence of metastasis.

Classified:	TO	Nlb	MO
	Tla	Nlb	MO
	T2a, T2b	NO, Nla, Nlb	MO

Stage III. A tumor larger than 5 cm with or without fixation or extension to fascia and chest wall; any amount of nodal involvement; no evidence of metastasis.

Classified:	Any T3	N1 or N2	MO

Stage IV. A tumor of any size with extension to chest wall and skin; any amount of nodal involvement; evidence of metastasis.

Classified:	T4	Any N	Any M
	Any T	N3	Any M
	Any T	Any N	M1

CANCER INFORMATION CENTERS

For information on other cancer-related subjects, call the toll-free number of the Cancer Information Service (CIS). Except for metropolitan Washington, D.C., and the states of Alaska and Hawaii, the offices of the Cancer Information Service are reached by a single toll-free long-distance line 1-800-4-CANCER (1-800-422-6237). Based on their area code, callers are automatically routed to the CIS office serving their area.

Only three of the nation's 21 Cancer Information Service offices do not share the new number. Their numbers are as follows:

- Alaska: 1-800-638-6070
- Hawaii: 1-808-524-1234
- Washington, D.C.: 1-202-636-5700

GLOSSARY

FOR A PHYSICIAN reading a medical journal or consulting with another colleague, medical terminology is a familiar part of communication. Consequently, it is natural for doctors to continue using technical language when speaking to patients, not realizing the confusion and anxiety they may cause. For the woman seeking information on breast cancer and breast reconstruction, it is a source of frustration. Before a woman is able to make an intelligent decision about breast reconstruction, she must be able to decipher the terminology. This glossary defines some of the more commonly used medical terms that women need to understand when consulting doctors about breast problems.

A

adjunctive (adjuvant) therapy. A secondary treatment in addition to the primary therapy. For example, chemotherapy is often used as an adjunctive therapy to a mastectomy.

adjuvant chemotherapy. After surgery, the use of anticancer drugs to prevent a recurrence of cancer. For women with breast cancer, the most important indicator for adjuvant chemotherapy is the spread of the cancer to the lymph nodes in the woman's undearm (axillary lymph nodes).

anterior axillary fold. Fold created where the breast and arm meet at the front of the armpit area. The large chest muscle (pectoralis major), which extends from the chest to the upper arm, is the main component of this fold.

areola. The circle of pigmented skin on the breast that surrounds the nipple.

aspirate. To remove or withdraw fluid from a cavity by applying suction.

augmentation mammoplasty (breast augmentation). An operation that enlarges a woman's breast, usually by placing a silicone breast implant behind the breast.

axilla. The underarm area behind the anterior axillary fold. It contains the axillary lymph nodes.

axillary dissection. Surgical removal of lymph nodes from the armpit. This tissue is then sent to the pathologist to determine if the breast cancer has spread.

B

benign. Opposite of cancerous, or malignant. A benign tumor is a noncancerous growth. It is self-limiting and does not spread to other areas of the body.

breast conserving surgery and irradiation. Treatment option for breast cancer whereby the tumor and axillary lymph nodes are surgically removed; most of the breast is preserved, and the remaining tissue is then treated by a course of irradiation.

breast implant. A soft, silicone form that can be placed in the body for simulation of a breast.

breast reconstruction. An operation to create a natural-looking breast shape after a mastectomy.

BSE. Breast self-examination. Self-inspection of the breasts by looking at them and feeling them.

C

cancer. A general term for the more than 100 diseases characterized by abnormal and uncontrolled growth of cells.

capsular contracture. A capsule or shell of scar tissue that may form around a woman's breast implant, giving it a feeling of firmness, as her body reacts to the implant.

chemotherapy. Treatment of cancer with anticancer drugs.

clavicle. Collarbone.

D

donor site. That part of the body from which tissue is taken for transfer to another part of the body for reconstruction.

E

edema. Excess fluid in the body, or a body part, that usually causes puffiness or swelling.

engorgement. An area of the body that is filled and stretched with fluid or distended with blood.

excisional biopsy. Surgical removal of tissue to be examined by opening the skin and removing the suspected tissue.

F

fascia. A sheet or broad band of fibrous or connective tissue that covers muscles and various organs of the body.

fibroadenoma. A benign, firm, identifiable breast tumor that commonly occurs in the breasts of young women.

fibrocystic disease. A benign breast condition, consisting of an overgrowth of fibrous tissue and the formation of cysts within the breast.

fibrous. Gristlelike strands of tough tissue that can grow in the body. For breast reconstruction, this usually refers to shell or scar tissue formation sometimes found around implants.

flap. A portion of tissue with its blood supply moved from one part of the body to another. Flaps of muscle and muscle, fat, and skin are frequently used to provide additional tissue for reconstructing a woman's breasts.

H

Halsted radical mastectomy. Surgical removal of the breast, skin, pectoralis muscles (both major and minor), all axillary lymph nodes, and fat for local treatment of a breast cancer.

hematoma. A collection of blood that can form in a wound after an injury or operation.

hormonal therapy. Treatment of cancer by alteration of the hormonal balance; some breast cancer cells will only grow in the presence of certain hormones.

I

in situ cancer. Localized or noninvasive cancer that has not begun to spread.

incisional biopsy. An operation to remove a portion of tissue that is suspected to be abnormal.

inert. Does not react or cause a reaction with something else.

infraclavicular nodes. Lymph nodes lying beneath the collarbone.

inframammary crease. The crease where a lower portion of the breast and chest wall meet.

invasive cancer. Cancer that has spread outside its site of origin to infiltrate and grow in surrounding tissue.

irradiation. A form of ionizing energy that can destroy or damage cells. Cancer cells tend to be more easily destroyed than the normal cells in the surrounding tissue. For breast cancer treatment, this therapy can be used with breast conserving surgery or as an adjunct to surgery to reduce the chance of cancer recurrence.

L

latissimus dorsi muscle. Triangular back muscle that, with some overlying skin, can be used as donor flap tissue for reconstructing a breast after mastectomy.

localized cancer. A cancer confined to its site of origin.

lumpectomy. Surgical removal of a cancerous tumor with or without a small margin of surrounding tissue.

lymph. Fluid that flows through the body, like blood, but in a separate system of vessels called the lymphatic system. Lymph fluid contains some waste products that are filtered through the lymph nodes and then this tissue fluid is returned to the blood.

lymph nodes. Structures in the lymphatic system that act as filters, catching bacteria and cancer cells, and contribute to the body's immune system, which fights disease.

M

malignant. Cancerous.

mammogram. A low-dose breast x-ray picture detailing the structure of breast tissue.

mammography. Process of taking breast x-ray pictures to detect breast cancer at an early stage.

mammoplasty. Breast operation to alter breast size.

mastectomy. Surgical removal of the breast, usually for treatment of cancer.

mastopexy. Breast lift to tighten the breast by removing sagging skin caused by the pull of gravity or the effects of aging.

menopause. The cessation of menstruation, usually as a result of aging. With this condition, a woman has a reduction in the level of female sex hormones present in her body.

metastasis. The spread of disease or cancer growths from one part of the body to another.

modified radical mastectomy. Surgical removal of the breast, some fat, and most of the lymph nodes in the armpit, leaving the chest wall muscles largely intact.

multicentric. More than one origin. Cancer cells may grow in several locations within the breasts and not be related to each other.

muscle flap. A muscle or portion of muscle that can be transferred with its blood supply to another part of the body for reconstructive purposes.

musculocutaneous (myocutaneous). Muscle and skin.

N

needle aspiration. Removal of fluid from a tumor or cyst with a small needle.

needle biopsy. Removal of a small sample of tissue with a wide-bore needle and suction.

nipple. The pigmented, central projection on the breast, containing the outer openings of the breast ducts.

nulliparous. Never having given birth to a child.

O

oncology. The study and treatment of tumors.

one-step procedure. Breast biopsy and mastectomy performed in a single operation.

P

palliative. Affording relief, but not cure, of symptoms such as pain.

palpable. Distinguishable by touch.

palpate. To feel.

palpation. Examining with the hand.

partial or segmental mastectomy. Breast surgery in which only a portion of the breast is removed, including the cancer and a surrounding margin of breast tissue.

pectoralis muscles. Muscular tissues attached to the front of the chest wall and extending to the upper arms. These are divided into the pectoralis major and pectoralis minor muscles. The pectoralis muscles usually are removed during a standard radical mastectomy, leaving a large deformity. They are preserved in a modified radical mastectomy.

pedicle. A connection of nourishing blood vessels from the body to a flap of tissue.

predisposition. A latent susceptibility to disease that may be activated under certain conditions.

primary. The first.

prophylactic mastectomy. Removal of high-risk breast tissue to prevent development of a cancer. This procedure usually is combined with breast reconstruction.

prosthesis. Any artificial body part. After a breast has been removed because of cancer, it is usually replaced by a breast-shaped form worn outside the body and fitting into the woman's brassiere in a specially designed pocket. Prostheses are made of different materials. For further information see Appendix C.

ptosis. Sagging breasts, usually the result of normal aging or changes produced from pregnancy, weight loss, or pull of gravity.

Q

quadrant mastectomy (quadrantectomy). Removal of one quarter of the breast.

R

radiation therapy (radiotherapy, radiation oncology). Treatment of disease by x-rays or other ionized energy.

radical mastectomy. Removal of the breast, underlying muscles, and underarm (axillary) lymph nodes.

reconstructive mammoplasty (breast reconstruction). Rebuilding of the breast by plastic surgical techniques.

rectus abdominis muscles. The vertical paired muscles on either side of the midline of the abdomen. These muscles can be used as donor tissue for breast reconstruction.

recurrence. Return of a tumor after the initial treatment of the primary tumor.

reduction mammoplasty. An operation for reducing the size of the breast by removing glandular and fatty tissue.

S

saline. Salt water; sometimes placed in breast implants.

seroma. A fluid mass caused by the localized accumulation of lymph fluid within a body part or area. This condition sometimes occurs after an operation. In breast surgery it may occur after an axillary dissection.

silicone. An inert chemical polymer that does not react with the body and is used to replace numerous body parts. Breast implants are made of silicone.

silicone gel. Silicone produced in a semisolid, semiliquid state and often used within breast implants; similar in consistency to a normal breast.

simple or total mastectomy. Removal of the breast only; lymph nodes and pectoralis muscles are preserved.

sloughing. The process in which the body rids itself of dead tissue. Frequently this happens when the tissue being used does not have an adequate blood supply.

subcutaneous mastectomy. Preventive mastectomy that removes most of the breast tissue but leaves the nipple intact.

survival rate. The percentage of people who live a period of time after a surgical procedure or the diagnosis of a disease as opposed to the percentage of those who die.

symmetry. Balance. When one side matches the other. One of the chief goals of the patient and plastic surgeon for breast reconstruction.

T

total mastectomy with axillary dissection. A mastectomy in which the breast tissue and most of the axillary lymph nodes are removed. Another name for modified radical mastectomy.

tumor. An abnormal growth of tissue.

two-step procedure. Breast biopsy and breast cancer treatment as two steps, allowing diagnosis of cancer and treatment to be separated by hours, days, or even longer periods of time.

X

x ray. High-energy radiation used in high doses to treat cancer or in low doses to diagnose the disease.

BIBLIOGRAPHY

THIS BIBLIOGRAPHY contains materials that we found helpful to us in preparing this book. Many of the pamphlets cited are available free through the National Cancer Institute. To allow our readers to explore these topics in whatever depth they feel is appropriate, we have included a mixture of articles and books; some are written for a general audience and others are written for a professional audience. Some books or pamphlets were particularly valuable to us, and these have been indicated with a black dot throughout the reference listings.

BREAST SELF-EXAMINATION

- Breast exams: what you should know, Pub. No. 82-2000, Washington, D.C., 1981, National Institutes of Health.

  Feldman, J.G.: Breast self-examination: relationship to stage of breast cancer at diagnosis, Cancer 47:2740, 1981.
- Foster, R. S., Jr., et al.: Breast self-examination practices and breast cancer stage, N. Engl. J. Med. 299:265, 1978.
- Foster, R. S., Jr., and Costanza, M.: Breast self-examination practices and breast cancer survival, Cancer 53:999, 1984.

  Greenwald, P., et al.: Estimated effect of breast self-examination and routine physician examinations on breast cancer mortality, N. Engl. J. Med. 299:271, 1978.
- How to examine your breasts, Pub. No. 2088-LE, New York, American Cancer Society.

  Milan, A. R.: Breast self-examination, New York, 1980, Liberty Publishing Co.

  Moore, F. D.: Breast self-examination, N. Engl. J. Med. 299:304, 1978.
- Myers, M. J.: Do-it-yourself breast testing, Health 14:18, Sept. 1982.

  Why now? Pub. No. 2039-LE, New York, 1980, American Cancer Society.

BREAST LUMPS AND BREAST CARE

Adcroft, P. G.: The breast disease that isn't cancer, Good Housekeeping, Aug. 1980.

Biopsy—diagnostic tool, Current Health 7:26, May 1981.

Black, S. T.: Specter of breast cancer: don't sit home and be afraid, McCall's, Feb. 1973.

Bland, K. L.: Analysis of breast cancer screening in women younger than fifty years, J.A.M.A. 245:1037, 1981.

Cancer screening and diagnosis: an annotated bibliography of public and patient education materials, Pub. No. 80-2153, Washington, D.C., 1980, National Institutes of Health.

Cohen, R.: Cancer may not be in lumps found in breast, St. Louis Post-Dispatch, Jan. 17, 1982.

Hunt, T. K.: Breast biopsies on outpatient surgeries, Surg. Gynecol. Obstet. 141:591, 1975.

Leis, H. P., Jr.: Diagnosis of breast cancer—basic factors, examination by the physician and breast self-examination, Professional Education Pub. No. 3402-PE, New York, American Cancer Society.

Leis, H. P., Jr.: Fibrocystic disease of the breast, J. Reprod. Med. 22:291, 1979.

Love, S. M., Gelman, R. S., and Silen, W.: Fibrocystic disease of the breast—a non-disease? N. Engl. J. Med. 307:1010, 1982.

Phillips, D., and Judd, R.: All about breasts, Ladies' Home Journal 99:88, 1982.

• Questions and answers about breast lumps, Pub. No. 83-2401, Washington, D.C., 1983, National Institutes of Health.

Robinson, D.: A better breast, Health 14:18, May 1982.

Rothenberg, R. E.: The complete book of breast care, New York, 1975, Crown Publishers, Inc.

BREAST CANCER INFORMATION

Breast cancer: annotated bibliography of public, patient and professional information and educational materials, Pub. No. 81-2002, Washington, D.C., 1980, National Institutes of Health.

Breast cancer: we're making progress every day, Pub. No. 82-2409, Washington, D.C., 1982, National Institutes of Health.

• The breast cancer digest: a guide to medical care, emotional support and educational programs, Pub. No. 84-1691, Baltimore, 1984, National Cancer Institute.

Cancer facts for women, Pub. No. 2007-LE, New York, 1982, American Cancer Society.

Cancer patient survival experience, Pub. No. 80-2148, Washington, D.C. 1980, National Institutes of Health.

Cancer screening and diagnosis — an annotated bibliography of public and patient education materials, Pub. No. 80-2153, Washington, D.C., 1980, National Institutes of Health.

• Coping with cancer: an annotated bibliography of public, patient and professional information and educational materials, Pub. No. 80-2129, Washington, D.C., 1980, National Institutes of Health.

• Coping with cancer: a resource for the health professional, Pub. No. 80-2080, Washington, D.C., 1980, National Institutes of Health.

• Coping with cancer update, Washington, D.C., 1983, National Institutes of Health.

Darion, E.: Exercises for mastectomy patients, McCall's 109:44, April 1982.

Eating hints: recipes and tips for better nutrition during cancer treatment, Pub. No. 83-2079, Washington, D.C., 1983, National Institutes of Health.

Gallager, H. S., Leis, H. P., Jr., Snyderman, R. V., and Urban, J. A., editors: The breast, St. Louis, 1978, The C. V. Mosby Co.

Good news about breast cancer, Harper's Bazaar 114:108, Sept. 1981.

Haiken, B. N.: A woman's guide to the breast — one in eleven, Largo, Fla., 1982, Bay Drive Publications.

If you've had breast cancer, Pub. No. 83-2400, Washington, D.C., 1983, National Institutes of Health.

Incidence and mortality in the United States, Natl. Cancer Inst. Monogr. 57:0, 1981.

McCauley, C. S.: Surviving breast cancer, New York, 1979, E. P. Dutton.

Miller, A. B.: Nutrition and cancer, Prev. Med. 9:189, 1980.

Moramarco, S. S.: Breast cancer: the news may be better than you think, Mademoiselle 88:94, March 1982.

National survey on breast cancer: a measure of progress in public understanding, Pub. No. 81-2306, Washington, D.C., 1980, National Institutes of Health.

Nutrition and the cancer patient: an annotated bibliography of patient and professional information and education materials, ed. 2, Pub. No. 82-1511, Washington, D.C., 1982, National Institutes of Health.

Patient rights: an annotated bibliography of cancer education materials for the public, patient, and professional, Pub. No. 81-2134, Washington, D.C., 1980, National Institutes of Health.

Rosenbaum, E. H.: Living with cancer, St. Louis, 1982, The C. V. Mosby Co.

Survival for cancer of the breast, Pub. No. 81-1542, Washington, D.C., 1981, National Institutes of Health.

Taking time: support for people with cancer and the people who care about them, Pub. No. 83-2059, Washington, D.C., 1983, National Institutes of Health.

Update breast cancer, Washington, D.C., 1983, National Institutes of Health.

What you need to know about cancer of the breast, Pub. No. 82-1556, Washington, D.C., 1982, National Institutes of Health.

PSYCHOLOGICAL ASPECTS OF BREAST CANCER

Ayalah, D., and Weinstock, I. J.: Breasts: women speak about their breasts and their lives, New York, 1979, Summit Books.

Bard, M., and Sutherland, A. M.: Psychological impact of cancer and its treatment: adaptation to radical mastectomy, IV. Cancer 8:656, 1955.

Bird, R. E.: Coming to terms with the fear of cancer, Los Angeles Times, July 17, 1980.

Brand, P. C., and Van Keep, P. A.: Breast cancer — psycho-social aspects of early detection and treatment, Baltimore, 1978, University Park Press.

Gold, M. A.: Causes of patients' delay in diseases of the breast, Cancer 17:564, 1964.

Holland, J.: Psychologic adaptation to breast cancer, Cancer 46(suppl. 4):1045, 1980.

Jobin, J.: How men respond to mastectomy, Woman's Day, Nov. 15, 1977.

May, H. J.: Psychosexual sequelae to mastectomy: implications for therapeutic and rehabilitative intervention, J. Rehabil. 46:29, Jan. 1980.

Meyerowitz, B. E.: The impact of mastectomy on the lives of women, Professional Psychology, Feb. 1981.

Morris, T.: Psychological and social adjustment to mastectomy, Cancer 40:2381, 1977.

My problem and how I solved it — I didn't feel like a real woman anymore, Good Housekeeping, 185:28, Sept. 1977.

Peck, A., and Boland, J.: Emotional reactions to radiation treatment, Cancer 40:180, 1977.

Polivy, J.: Psychological effects of mastectomy on a woman's feminine self-concept, J. Nerv. Ment. Dis. 164:77, Feb. 1977.

Psychologic aspects of cancer — Jan. 1978 through July 1981, Literature Search No. 81-18, Washington, D.C., National Library Of Medicine.

The psychological impact of cancer, Professional Education Pub. No. 3009-P.E., New York, American Cancer Society.

Schain, W. S.: Sexual problems of patients with cancer. In De Vita, V. Hellman, S., and Rosenberg, S., editors: Cancer: principles and practices of oncology, Philadelphia, 1982, J. B. Lippincott Co.

Schottenfeld, D., and Robbins, G. F.: Quality of survival among patients who have had radical mastectomy, Cancer 26:650, 1970.

Wellish, D. K.: Psychosocial aspects of mastectomy: the man's perspective, Am. J. Psychiatry, May 1978.

Witkin, M. H.: Sex therapy and mastectomy, J. Sex Marital Ther. 1:290, 1975.

Women's attitudes regarding breast cancer, New York, 1973 Gallup Organization, Inc.

PERSONAL ACCOUNTS OF BREAST CANCER AND RECONSTRUCTION

Armel, P.: After mastectomy: choosing to look different, Ms., p. 22, July 1981.

DiSimone, M. A.: A genuine smile — one woman's personal accounting of mastectomy and breast reconstruction, Avon Park, Fla., 1982, The Vin Mar Agency, Inc.

Ford, B.: The times of my life, New York, 1978, Harper & Row, Publishers, Inc.

Kushner, R.: Why me? What every woman should know about breast cancer to save her life, New York, 1977, New American Library, Inc.

Kushner, R.: My side, Working Woman 8:160, May 1983.

Lake, A.: An honest report on breast cancer, Redbook 157:65, Sept. 1981.

Lamberg, L.: Back to business: surviving the biggest crisis of all, Working Woman 6:85, April 1981.

Pepper, C.B.: The victors — patients who conquered cancer, The New York Times, Jan. 29, 1984.

Rollin, B.: First you cry, Philadelphia, 1976, J. B. Lippincott Co.

• Shapero, L., and Goodman, A.: Never say die: a doctor and patient talk about breast cancer, New York, 1980, Appleton-Century-Crofts.

Snyder, M. B.: Breast reconstruction — new hope after mastectomy, Woman's Day, p. 40, Oct. 25, 1983.

Zalon, J.: I am whole again: the case for breast reconstruction after mastectomy, New York, 1978, Random House, Inc.

BREAST CANCER TREATMENT OPTIONS

Bedwani, R.: Management and survival of patients with "minimal" breast cancer, Cancer 47:2769, 1981.

Bedwinek, J.: Treatment of stage I and II adenocarcinoma of the breast by tumor excision and irradiation, Int. J. Radiat. Oncol. Biol. Phys. 7:1553, 1981.

• Bedwinek, J.: Breast cancer: primary treatment. In Gilbert, H., editor: Modern radiation oncology: classic literature and current management, vol. 2, Philadelphia, 1984, Harper & Row, Publishers.

Bonadonna, G.: Dose effect of adjuvant chemotherapy in breast cancer, N. Engl. J. Med. 304:10, 1981.

• Brody, J. E.: Cancer therapies improve, New York Times, April 15, 1981.

• Breast cancer: A measure of progress in public understanding, Pub. No. 81-2291, Washington, D.C., 1980, National Institutes of Health.

• Breast cancer: the retreat from radical surgery, Consumer Reports 46:24, Jan. 1981.

Breast cancer resource guide. I. Washington, D.C., 1980, National Women's Health Network.

Breast saving surgery—radiation for early cancer gaining advocates, J.A.M.A. **245**:661, 1981.

Cancer treatment: An annotated bibliography of patient materials, Pub. No. 81-2152, Washington, D.C., 1981, National Institutes of Health.

Carter, S. K.: Chemotherapy of cancer, New York, 1981, John Wiley & Sons, Inc.

• Chemotherapy and you: a guide to self-help during treatment, Pub. No. 83-1136, Washington, D.C., 1983, National Institutes of Health.

DeVita, V.: Cancer treatment: medicine for the layman, Pub. No. 82-1807, Washington, D.C., 1982, National Institutes of Health.

Final word on disputed mastectomies, Science **202**:728, 1978.

Fisher, B.: The evolution of breast cancer surgery: past, present, and future, Semin. Oncol. **5**:386, 1978.

Fisher, B., et al.: Comparison of radical mastectomy with alternative treatments for primary breast cancer: a first report of results from a prospective randomized clinical trial, Cancer **39**:2827, 1977.

Good news about breast cancer, Harper's Bazaar **114**:108, Sept. 1981.

Goodson, W. H., III: Diagnosing the data on the treatment of stage I and stage II breast cancer, Resident and Staff Physician Sept. 1982, p. 63.

• Harris, J. R., Hellman, S., and Silen, W.: Conservative management of breast cancer: new surgical and radiotherapeutic techniques, Philadelphia, 1983, J. B. Lippincott Co.

Lake, A.: An honest report on breast cancer, Redbook **157**:65, Sept. 1981.

Maddox, W. A., et al.: A randomized prospective trial of radical (Halsted) mastectomy versus modified radical mastectomy in 311 breast cancer patients, Ann. Surg. **198**:207, 1983.

Medicine for the layman: cancer treatment, Pub. No. 82-1807, Washington, D.C., 1982, National Institutes of Health.

Montague, E. C., et al.: Conservation surgery and irradiation for the treatment of favorable breast cancer, Cancer **43**:1058, 1979.

• Morra, M., and Pots, E.: Choices: realistic alternatives in cancer treatment, New York, 1980, Avon Books.

Packard, R. A., Prosnitz, L. R., and Bobrow, S. N.: Selection of breast cancer patients for adjuvant chemotherapy, J.A.M.A. **238**:1034, 1977.

• Radiation therapy and you: a guide to self-help during treatment, Pub. No. 83-2227, Washington, D.C., 1982, National Institutes of Health.

Rebuke for radical mastectomy, Time **118**:63, July 13, 1981.

Schain, W. S., Edwards, B. E., Garrell, C. R., et al.: Psychosocial and physical outcomes of primary breast cancer therapy: mastectomy versus excisional biopsy and irradiation, Breast Cancer Res. Treat. **3**:377, 1983.

• Spear, R.: Breast cancer—new research, new options, New York, Jan. 16, 1984, p. 24.

Spletter, M. A.: A woman's choice: New options in the treatment of breast cancer, Boston, 1982, Beacon Press.

Veronesi, U.: Comparing radical mastectomy with quadrantectomy, axillary dissection and radiotherapy in patients with small cancers of the breast, N. Engl. J. Med. 305:6, 1981.

PREVENTIVE (PROPHYLACTIC) MASTECTOMY FOR THE WOMAN AT RISK

Anderson, D. E.: Genetic study of breast cancer: identification of a high risk group, Cancer 34:1090, 1974.

Anderson, D. E.: Breast cancer in families, Cancer 40:1855, 1977.

Berman, C.: Breast surgery to prevent cancer: the big dispute, Good Housekeeping 192:151, March 1981.

Breast cancer — some trying surgery as a preventive, Los Angeles Times, Dec. 9, 1980.

Buchler, P.: Patient selection for prophylactic mastectomy: Who is at high risk? Plast. Reconstr. Surg. 72:324, 1983.

Clark, M., and Shapiro, D.: Breast surgery before cancer, Newsweek 96:100, Dec. 1, 1980.

Dowden, R. V.: Total mastectomy for premalignant disease with immediate reconstruction. In Gant, T. D., and Vasconez, L., editors: Postmastectomy reconstruction, Baltimore, 1981, Williams & Wilkins.

Goldwyn, R. M.: Subcutaneous mastectomy, N. Engl. J. Med. 297:503, 1977.

Jarrett, J. R., Cutler, R. G., and Teal, D. F.: Subcutaneous mastectomy in small, large or ptotic breasts with immediate submuscular placement of implants, Plast. Reconstr. Surg. 62:381, 1978.

Kelly, P. T.: Refinements in breast cancer risk analysis, Arch. Surg. 116:364, March 1981.

Leis, H. P., Jr.: Epidemiology of breast cancer: identification of the high risk woman. In Gallagher, H. S., Leis, H. P., Jr., Snyderman, R. V., and Urban, J. A., editors: The breast, St. Louis, 1978, The C. V. Mosby Co.

Love, S.: Discussion of patient selection for prophylactic mastectomy: Who is at high risk? Plast. Reconstr. Surg. 72:326, 1983.

Peacock, E.: Biological basis for management of benign disease of the breast: the case against subcutaneous mastectomy, Plast. Reconstr. Surg. 55:14, 1975.

BREAST RECONSTRUCTION

Apfelberg, D. B., Laub, D. R., Maser, M. R., and Lash, H.: Submuscular breast reconstruction — indications and techniques, Ann. Plast. Surg. 7:213, 1981.

Berkowitch, S.: Psychological results of reconstructed patients, Acta Chir. Belg. 79(2):165, 1980.

A better breast—mastectomy patients get a new bust and a bonus "tummy tuck," Health 14:18, May 1982.

Bosnak, S.: Reconstruction eases horror of mastectomy, Journal Herald, Dayton, Ohio, Oct. 2, 1978.

• Bostwick, J. III: Aesthetic and reconstructive breast surgery, St. Louis, 1983, The C. V. Mosby Co.

Bostwick, J. III: Breast reconstruction after radical mastectomy, Plast. Reconstr. Surg. 61:682, 1978.

Bostwick, J. III: Sixty latissimus dorsi flaps, Plast. Reconstr. Surg. 63:113, 1978.

Brent, B., and Bostwick, J. III: Nipple-areola reconstruction with auricular tissues, Plast. Reconstr. Surg. 60:353, 1977.

Breast building—mastectomy with a bonus tuck, Time 118:49, Nov. 2, 1981.

• Breast reconstruction, New York, 1982, American Cancer Society. (Slide presentation available for viewing through local and regional chapters.)

• Breast reconstruction—creating a new breast contour after mastectomy, Pub. No. 81-2151, Washington, D.C., 1980, National Institutes of Health.

• Breast reconstruction following mastectomy for cancer—some questions and answers, Pub. No. 4574-P.S., Chicago, 1979, American Society of Plastic and Reconstructive Surgeons.

Broadbent, T. R., Metz, P. S., and Woolf, R. M.: Restoring the mammary areola by a skin graft from the upper inner thigh, Br. J. Plast. Surg. 30:220, 1977.

Clifford, E.: The reconstruction experience: the search for restitution. In Georgiade, N. G., editor: Breast reconstruction following mastectomy, St. Louis, 1979, The C. V. Mosby Co.

Clifford, E.: Breast reconstruction following mastectomy: social characteristics of patients seeking the procedure. I. Ann. Plast. Surg. 5:341, 1980.

Clifford, E.: Breast reconstruction following mastectomy: marital characteristics of patients seeking the procedure. II. Ann. Plast. Surg. 5:344, 1980.

Dowden, R. V.: Advising the mastectomy patient about reconstruction, Am. Fam. Physician 19(5):103, 1979.

Goin, J. M., and Goin, M. K.: Changing the body: psychological effects of plastic surgery, Baltimore, 1981, Williams & Wilkins.

Goin, M. K., and Goin, J. M.: Midlife reactions to mastectomy and subsequent breast reconstruction, Arch. Gen. Psychiatry 38:225, 1981.

Goin, M. K., and Goin, J. M.: Psychological reactions to prophylactic mastectomy synchronous with contralateral breast reconstruction, Plast. Reconstr. Surg. 70:355, 1982.

Goin, M. C.: Discussion—the psychological impact of immediate breast reconstruction for women with early breast cancer, Plast. Reconstr. Surg. 73:627, 1984.

Goldwyn, R. M.: Consultation for breast reconstruction (editorial), Plast. Reconstr. Surg. **73**:818, 1984.

Hartrampf, C. R., Scheflan, M., and Black, P. W.: Breast reconstruction following mastectomy with a transverse abdominal island flap: anatomical and clinical observations, Plast. Reconstr. Surg. **69**:216, 1982.

• Levinson, J.: Breast reconstruction: a patient's view, Plast. Reconstr. Surg. **73**:703, 1984.

Mathes, S. J., and Nahai, F., editors: Clinical applications for muscle and musculocutaneous flaps, St. Louis, 1982, The C. V. Mosby Co.

Noone, R. B., Frazier, T. B., Hayward, C. Z., and Skiles, M. S.: Patient acceptance of immediate reconstruction following mastectomy, Plast. Reconstr. Surg. **69**:632, 1982.

Plastic Surgery: post-op care that pays off, Harper's Bazaar 115:149, 1982.

Schain, W. S.: Reconstructive mammoplasty: reversibility of a trauma. In Western States Conference on cancer rehabilitation, Palo Alto, Calif., 1982, Bull Publishing Co.

Schain, W. S., Jacobs, E., and Wellisch, D. K.: Psychosocial issues in breast reconstruction: intrapsychic, interpersonal, and practical concerns, Clin. Plast. Surg. **2**:237, 1984.

Schain, W. S., et al.: The sooner the better: a study of psychological factors of women undergoing immediate versus delayed breast reconstruction, submitted for publication.

Stevens, L. A., et al.: The psychological impact of immediate breast reconstruction for women with early breast cancer, Plast. Reconstr. Surg. **73**:619, 1984.

Teimourian, B., and Adham, M. N.: Survey of patients' responses to breast reconstruction, Ann. Plast. Surg. **9**:321, 1982.

• Zalon, J.: I am whole again: the case for breast reconstruction after mastectomy, New York, 1978, Random House, Inc.

Index